Cardiovascular Trials Review

Second Edition

Edited by:

Yochai Birnbaum, MD
Robert A. Kloner, MD, PhD

Studies Compiled By:

Robert A. Kloner, MD, PhD
Yochai Birnbaum, MD

Yochai Birnbaum, MD
Research Fellow in Cardiology,
Cedars Sinai Medical Center,
Los Angeles, CA

Robert A. Kloner, MD, PhD
Director of Research,
Heart Institute,
Good Samaritan Hospital,
Professor of Medicine,
University of Southern California,
Los Angeles, CA

ISBN 0-9626020-6X

Printed in the United States of America

Table of Contents:

I. Acute Myocardial Infarction
a. Thrombolytic Therapy

f. Miscellaneous

2. Unstable Angina

3. Stable Angina Pectoris and Silent Ischemia-Medical Therapy

4. Interventional Cardiology

a. PTCA or CABG Versus Medical Therapy

b. PTCA Versus CABG.

c. PTCA Versus Other Percutaneous Devices

d. Medical Therapy to Prevent Restenosis After Intracoronary Interventions or Occlusion After Coronary Artery Bypass Grafting

5. Hypertension

6. Congestive Heart Failure (CHF) and CHF with Arrhythmia

10. Coronary Artery Disease, Atherosclerosis- Prevention of Progression

11. Ongoing Clinical Trials

Introduction

The purpose of *Cardiovascular Trials Review Second Edtion* is to review those trials which have made a major impact on the practice of clinical cardiology within the last six years. We have included only studies that were published in English and concentrated mainly on publications that have appeared since 1990 and have studied either pharmacological or device therapy. The text is divided into major headings of diseases such as myocardial infarction and unstable angina. In general, we gave priority to prospective randomized trials with preference to multicenter studies and those that included several hundred patients. In this second edition we have added over 50 new studies and concentrated on trials from 1996-1997.

Unfortunately, we were not able to include all studies. There are many other excellent studies which may not appear in this review. However, a review of the trials included in this book should give the reader a flavor of the types and designs of major clinical trials that have influenced the practice of clinical cardiology.

We have tried to use only minimal amount of abbreviations in the text: CI- confidence interval; ECG- electrocardiogram; and RR- relative risk.

The drugs, indications for drugs, and drug dosages may or may not be approved for general use by the Food and Drug Administration (FDA). Physicians should consult the package inserts and/or Physicians' Desk Reference for drug indications, contraidications, side effects and dosages as recommended. We thank Sharon L. Hale for her help with this manuscript.

Robert A. Kloner, MD, PhD
Yochai Birnbaum, MD
Los Angeles, CA
March, 1997.

1. Acute Myocardial Infarction

a. Thrombolytic Therapy

GISSI

Gruppo Italiano per lo Studio della Streptochinasi nell'Infarto miocardico

Title	a. Effectiveness of intravenous thrombolytic treatment in acute myocardial infarction. b. Long-term effects of intravenous thrombolysis in acute myocardial infarction: final report of the GISSI study.
Authors	GISSI
Reference	a. Lancet 1986;I:397-401. b. Lancet 1987;II:871-874.
Disease	Acute myocardial infarction.
Purpose	To evaluate the efficacy of intravenous streptokinase to reduce in-hospital and 1-year mortality in patients with acute myocardial infarction, and to define the time interval from onset of symptoms to therapy that therapy is still effective.
Design	Randomized, open label, multicenter.
Patients	11,712 patients with suspected acute myocardial infarction ≤12 h of onset of symptoms, with ≥1 mm ST elevation or depression in any limb lead or ≥2 mm in any precordial lead. No age restriction.
Follow-up	1 year.
Treatment regimen	Streptokinase 1.5 million U IV over 1 h, or no treatment.
Additional therapy	According to normal practice. No restrictions.

Gruppo Italiano per lo Studio della Streptochinasi nell'Infarto miocardico

(continued)

Results

a. 21 day course: Overall mortality was 13.0% in the control and 10.7% in the treated group (relative risk 0.81, 95% CI 0.72-0.90,p=0.0002). In patients treated within 3 h from onset of symptoms mortality was 12.0% and 9.2% for the control and streptokinase groups (RR 0.74, 95% CI 0.63-0.87, p=0.0005), while for those treated 3-6 h the mortality was 14.1% and 11.7%, respectively (RR 0.80, 95% CI 0.66-0.98, p=0.03). Treatment beyond 6 h did not result in a significant difference in mortality between the groups (14.1% vs 12.6%, p=NS, RR 0.87 for those treated 6-9 h; and 13.6% vs 15.8%, p=NS, RR 1.19 for those treated 9-12 h after onset of symptoms). Subgroup analysis revealed beneficial effects for streptokinase in patients with anterior and multi-site infarction. However, patients with lateral infarctions or ST depression had a trend towards worse outcome with streptokinase than without (although without statistical significance). The incidence of anaphylactic shock and bleeding attributed to streptokinase were low.
b. After 1 year mortality was 17.2% in the streptokinase and 19.0% in the control group (RR 0.90, 95% CI 0.84-0.97, p=0.008). The difference in mortality was seen only in those treated within 6 h of onset of symptoms.

Conclusions

a. Streptokinase is a safe and effective therapy for patients with acute myocardial infarction treated within 6 h of onset of symptoms.
b. The beneficial effects of streptokinase were still apparent after 1 year.

TIMI-1

Thrombolysis in Myocardial Infarction Trial (phase 1)

Title	Thrombolysis in Myocardial Infarction (TIMI) Trial, phase I: a comparison between intravenous tissue plasminogen activator and intravenous streptokinase. Clinical findings through hospital discharge.
Authors	Chesbero JH, Knatterud G, Roberts R, et al.
Reference	Circulation 1987;76:142-154.
Disease	Acute myocardial infarction.
Purpose	To compare two regimens of intravenous thrombolytic therapy: rt-PA and streptokinase.
Design	Randomized, double blind, multicenter.
Patients	290 patients with acute myocardial infarction <75 years old < 7 hours from onset of symptoms with chest pain>30 min and ST elevation ≥0.1 mV in ≥2 contiguous leads. Patients with cardiogenic shock were excluded.
Follow-up	Coronary angiography before and 10, 20, 30, 45, 60, 75, 90 min, after onset of thrombolytic therapy and predischarge. Clinical visits at six weeks and six months
Treatment regimen	Streptokinase 1.5 million units or placebo IV over 1 h, and rt-PA or placebo over 3 h (40, 20, and 20 mg in the first, second and third hours).
Additional therapy	Lidocaine (1-1.5 mg/kg bolus + infusion 2-4 μg/min) for >24 h; intracoronary nitroglycerin 200 μg; heparin 5000 U bolus and infusion 1000 U/h for 8-10 days. Aspirin 325 mg X3/d and dipyridamole 75 mg X3/d after heparin was stopped.

TIMI-1

Thrombolysis in Myocardial Infarction Trial (phase 1)

(continued)

Results

At 30 min after initiation of therapy 24% and 8% of the rt-PA and streptokinase -treated patients achieved TIMI grade flow of 2 or 3 (P<0.001). At 90 min after initiation of therapy, 62% of the rt-PA and 31% of the streptokinase-treated patients achieved TIMI grade flow of 2 or 3 (P<0.001). 44% and 22% of the rt-PA and streptokinase-treated patients had patent arteries upon discharge (p<0.001). There was no difference in global or regional left ventricular function either in the pre-treatment or predischarge study. Fever or chills occurred in 4% and 15% of the rt-PA and streptokinase groups (p<0.01). Death within 21 days occurred in 4% and 5% of the rt-PA and streptokinase groups. The reduction in circulating fibrinogen and plasminogen and the increase in plasma fibrin split products at 3 and 24 h were significantly more pronounced in the streptokinase treated patients (p<0.001). The occurrence of bleeding was comparable in the 2 groups (66% and 67% of the rt-PA and streptokinase, respectively).

Conclusions

Treatment with rt-PA resulted in more rapid reperfusion than streptokinase. However, there was no difference in either mortality, bleeding complications or left ventricular function between the groups.

ISIS-2

International Study of Infarct Survival 2

Title	Randomized trial of intravenous streptokinase, oral aspirin, both, or neither among 17,187 cases of suspected acute myocardial infarction: ISIS-2.
Authors	ISIS-2 Collaborative Group.
Reference	Lancet 1988;II:349-360.
Disease	Acute myocardial infarction.
Purpose	To assess the efficacy of oral aspirin, streptokinase infusion, and their combination in the treatment of acute myocardial infarction.
Design	Randomized, double blind, 2X2 factorial, placebo-controlled, multicenter.
Patients	17,187 patients with suspected acute myocardial infarction <24 h of onset of symptoms.
Follow-up	Maximum 34 months, median 15 months.
Treatment regimen	1. Streptokinase 1.5 million U over 1 h IV. 2. Aspirin 162.5 mg/d for 1 month. 3. Streptokinase 1.5 million U over 1 h IV + Aspirin 162.5 mg/d for 1 month. 4. Neither.
Additional therapy	No restrictions.

Results

5-week vascular mortality among the streptokinase and placebo treated patients was 9.2% and 12.0%, respectively (odds reduction: 25%, 95% CI 18-32%, $p<0.00001$). 5-week vascular mortality among the aspirin treated was 9.4% and for the placebo 11.8% (odds reduction: 23%, 95% CI 15-30%, $p<0.00001$). The combination of aspirin and streptokinase was better than either agent alone. 5-week vascular mortality among the streptokinase and aspirin treated patients was 8.0%, while it was 13.2% among those allocated to neither treatment (odds reduction: 42%, 95% CI: 34-50%). The odds reductions at treatment 0-4, 5-12, and 13-24 h after onset of symptoms were 35%, 16%, and 21% for streptokinase alone; 25%, 21%, and 21% for aspirin alone; and 53%, 32%, and 38% for the combination. Streptokinase was associated with excess bleeding requiring transfusion (0.5% vs 0.2%, $p<0.001$), and of cerebral hemorrhage (0.1% vs 0.0%, $p<0.02$). However, total strokes were similar (0.7% vs 0.8%). Aspirin reduced the rates of non-fatal reinfarction (1.0% vs 2.0%, $p<0.00001$) and non-fatal stroke (0.3% vs 0.6%, $p<0.01$) and was not associated with increased risk of cerebral or non-cranial hemorrhages. Patients allocated to the combination therapy had fewer reinfarctions (1.8% vs 2.9%), strokes (0.6% vs 1.1%), and deaths (8.0% vs 13.2%) than those allocated to neither therapy. The difference in mortality produced by either aspirin, streptokinase, or their combination remained significant after 15 months of follow-up.

Conclusions

Aspirin and streptokinase independently reduced mortality in patients with acute myocardial infarction. The combination of the two drugs has a synergistic effect on mortality without increasing the rates of stroke.

AIMS

APSAC Intervention Mortality Study

Title	a. Effect of intravenous APSAC on mortality after acute myocardial infarction: preliminary report of a placebo-controlled clinical trial. b. Long-term effects of intravenous anistreplase in acute myocardial infarction: final report of the AIMS study.
Authors	AIMS Trial Study Group.
Reference	a. Lancet 1988;I;545-549. b. Lancet 1990;335:427-431.
Disease	Acute myocardial infarction.
Purpose	To compare survival up to 1 year in patients with acute myocardial infarction randomized to APSAC (anisoylated plasminogen streptokinase activator complex) or placebo.
Design	Randomized, double blind, placebo-controlled, multicenter.
Patients	a. 1004 patients, age ≤70 years with acute myocardial infarction, ≥30 min pain, <6 h of onset of symptoms, ≥1 mm ST elevation in ≥2 limb leads or >2 mm in >2 precordial leads. b. 1258 patients, same criteria, including the first 1004 patients.
Follow-up	1 year.
Treatment regimen	APSAC 30 U or placebo IV over 5 min.
Additional therapy	IV heparin started 6 h after initiation of therapy, warfarin for ≥3 months. Other medications according to common practice. Timolol 10 mg/d for 1 year if not contraindicated.

AIMS

APSAC Intervention Mortality Study

(continued)

Results

a. 30-day mortality was 12.2% on placebo and 6.4% on APSAC (47% reduction of mortality, 95% CI 21-65%, p=0.0016). Percentage reduction of mortality with APSAC was similar whether therapy was started 0-4 or 4-6 h after onset of symptoms.
b. 30-day mortality was 12.1% on placebo and 6.4% on APSAC (50.5% reduction of mortality, 95% CI 26-67%, p=0.0006). 1 year mortality was 17.8% on placebo and 11.1% on APSAC (42.7% reduction of mortality, 95% CI 21-59%, p=0.0007). Major cardiovascular complications (shock, cardiac arrest, rupture, ventricular septal defect, and ventricular fibrillation) occurred in 12.3% and 16.7% of the APSAC and placebo groups, respectively (p=0.03).

Conclusions

Intravenous APSAC within 6 h of onset of symptoms reduced mortality in acute myocardial infarction.

ASSET

Anglo-Scandinavian Study of Early Thrombolysis

Title	a. Trial of tissue plasminogen activator for mortality reduction in acute myocardial infarction. Anglo-Scandinavian Study of early Thrombolysis (ASSET). b. Effects of alteplase in acute myocardial infarction: 6-month results from the ASSET study.
Authors	Wilcox RG, von der Lippe G, Olsson CG, et al.
Reference	a. Lancet 1988;II:525-530. b. Lancet 1990;335:1175-1178.
Disease	Acute myocardial infarction.
Purpose	To evaluate the efficacy of tissue plasminogen activator versus placebo in reduction of mortality in acute myocardial infarction.
Design	Randomized, double blind, placebo-controlled, multicenter.
Patients	a. 5009 patients, b. 5013 patients, age 18-75 years, with suspected acute myocardial infarction within 5 h of onset of symptoms. No ECG criteria were required.
Follow-up	6 months.
Treatment regimen	Tissue plasminogen activator (t-PA) or placebo 10 mg IV bolus, 50 mg infusion over 1 h, and then 40 mg over 2 h.
Additional therapy	IV heparin 5000 U bolus, and infusion of 1000 U/h for 21 h.

ASSET

Anglo-Scandinavian Study of Early Thrombolysis

(continued)

Results

a. One month mortality was 7.2% and 9.8%, in the t-PA and placebo groups (a relative reduction of 26%, 95% CI 11-39%, p=0.0011). Bleeding (major+minor) and major bleeding occurred in 6.3% and 1.4% of the t-PA, and 0.8% and 0.4% of the placebo groups, respectively. The incidence of stroke was similar (1.1% and 1.0%). There was no difference in recurrent infarction or development of heart failure rates. In those with abnormal ECG on entry, t-PA was associated with 24.5% relative reduction in 1 month mortality (8.5% vs 11.2%, 95% CI 9-37%).
b. 6 month mortality rate was 10.4% in the t-PA and 13.1% in the placebo group (relative reduction of risk 21%, 95% CI 8-32%, p=0.0026). 6 month mortality for patients with proven infarction was 12.6% and 17.1%, respectively (relative reduction of risk 26.3%, 95% CI 14-38%). The effect was similar for anterior and inferior infarctions. However, t-PA did not reduce cardiac readmissions, reinfarctions, development of neart failure, angina, or death beyond 1 month. 12 month mortality (for 4230 patients) was 13.2% and 15.1% for t-PA and placebo group (p<0.05).

Conclusions

t-PA therapy within 5 h of onset of symptoms, compared to placebo, reduced mortality sustained to 1 year, but not the rates of recurrent infarction, angina or development of heart failure.

GISSI-2

Gruppo Italiano per lo Studio della Streptochinasi nell'Infarto miocardico 2

Title	a. GISSI-2: A factorial randomized trial of alteplase versus streptokinase and heparin versus no heparin among 12,490 patients with acute myocardial infarction. b. In-hospital mortality and clinical course of 20,891 patients with suspected acute myocardial infarction randomized between alteplase and streptokinase with or without heparin.
Authors	a. GISSI b. The International Study Group.
Reference	a. Lancet 1990;336:65-71. b. Lancet 1990;336:71-75.
Disease	Acute myocardial infarction.
Purpose	To compare the efficacy of intravenous streptokinase and tissue plasminogen activator (t-PA) for the treatment of acute myocardial infarction, and to evaluate the effects of adding heparin therapy to aspirin on the incidence of recurrent ischemia.
Design	Randomized, open label, 2X2 factorial, multicenter.
Patients	a. 12,381 patients. b. 20,768 patients (including 12,490 from the GISSI-2). All patients had chest pain + ST elevation ≥1mm in any limb lead and/or ST≥2 mm in any precordial lead, within 6 h of onset of symptoms. No age limit.
Follow-up	In-hospital course, predischarge echocardiography.

GISSI-2

Gruppo Italiano per lo Studio della Streptochinasi nell'Infarto miocardico 2

(continued)

Treatment regimen

a. Streptokinase 1.5 million U over 30-60 min + heparin SC 12,500 UX2/d, starting 12 h after initiation of thrombolytic infusion and continued until discharge.
b. t-PA 10 mg bolus, 50 mg over 1 h, and 40 mg over 2 h + heparin SC 12,500 UX2/d, starting 12 h after initiation of thrombolytic infusion and continued until discharge.
c. Streptokinase 1.5 million U over 30-60 min without heparin.
d. t-PA 10 mg bolus, 50 mg over 1 h, and 40 mg over 2 h without heparin.

Additional therapy

Oral aspirin 300-325 mg/d. Atenolol 5-10 mg IV.

Results

a. The t-PA and streptokinase groups did not differ in mortality (9.0% and 8.6%), clinical heart failure (7.7% and 8.1%), or occurrence of left ventricular ejection fraction ≤35% (2.5% and 2.2%). Combined end points occurred in 23.1% and 22.5%, respectively. The rates of recurrent infarction, post-infarction angina, stroke, and bleeding were not different between the t-PA and streptokinase groups. Allergic reactions and hypotension were more common in the streptokinase than t-PA treated patients. There was no differences regarding mortality (8.3% vs 9.3%), heart failure (8.0% vs 7.8%), ejection fraction ≤35% (2.3% vs 2.4%) between the heparin and no-heparin groups. There was no difference in reinfarction, post-infarction angina, and stroke between the two groups. Major bleeding was more common in the heparin treated patients (1.0% vs 0.6%, RR 1.64, 95% CI 1.09-2.45).
b. In-hospital mortality was 8.9% for t-PA and 8.5% for streptokinase (RR 1.05, 95% CI 0.96-1.16), and 8.5% for heparin versus 8.9% without heparin. More strokes occurred with t-PA (1.3%) than with streptokinase (0.9%), while major bleeding occurred in 0.6% and 0.9% of the t-PA and streptokinase treated patients.

Conclusions

Streptokinase and t-PA appear equally effective and safe. Adding heparin subcutaneously to thrombolysis and aspirin did not alter prognosis, except for an increase in major bleeding.

MITI-1

Myocardial Infarction Triage and Intervention

Title	Myocardial infarction triage and intervention project- phase I: patient characteristics and feasibility of prehospital initiation of thrombolytic therapy.
Authors	Weaver WD, Eisenberg MS, Martin JS, et al.
Reference	J Am Coll Cardiol 1990;15:925-931.
Disease	Acute myocardial infarction.
Purpose	To assess the feasibility and the time saving, of the strategy of prehospital initiation of thrombolytic therapy by paramedics.
Design	Patients with chest pain were evaluated by paramedics by obtaining history, physical examination, and electrocardiogram that was transmitted to a base station physician. The physician determined whether the patient met the criteria for prehospital thrombolysis.
Patients	2472 patients, <75 years old, with chest pain ≥15 min and <6 h, who called 911.
Follow-up	9 months.

Results

677 patients (27%) had suitable clinical findings consistent with possible acute myocardial infarction and no apparent risk for thrombolytic therapy. Electrocardiograms of 522 of the 677 patients were transmitted to the base station. Only 107 (21%) of these tracings demonstrated ST elevation. 453 patients developed acute myocardial infarction in hospital. 163 (36%) of the 453 patients met the screening history and examination criteria and 105 (23.9%) had ST elevation. The average time from onset of symptoms to prehospital diagnosis was 72±52 min (median 52 min). This was 73±44 min (median 62 min) earlier than the actual time when thrombolytic therapy was started in hospital.

Conclusions

Paramedic selection of patients for potential prehospital initiation of thrombolytic therapy is feasible and may shorten the time to initiation of thrombolytic therapy.

TEAM-2

The Second Thrombolytic Trial of Eminase in Acute Myocardial Infarction

Title	Multicenter patency trial of intravenous anistreplase compared with streptokinase in acute myocardial infarction.
Authors	Anderson JL, Sorensen SG, Moreno FL, et al.
Reference	Circulation 1991;83;126-140.
Disease	Acute myocardial infarction.
Purpose	To compare the efficacy of anistreplase (APSAC) and streptokinase on early patency and reocclusion rates.
Design	Randomized, double blind, multicenter.
Patients	370 patients, aged <76 years, with chest pain of >30 min, ≤4 h of onset of symptoms, and ST elevation of ≥1 mm in ≥1 limb lead or ≥2 mm in ≥1 precordial lead. Patients in cardiogenic shock, previous coronary artery bypass grafting, balloon angioplasty within 1 month, blood pressure >200/120 mmHg, or contraindications to thrombolytic therapy were excluded.
Follow-up	90-240 min coronary angiography. Patients with TIMI flow 0 or 1 were allowed to undergo angioplasty. Patients with initial TIMI flow 2-3, who did not undergo mechanical intervention, were catheterized again 18-48 h after initiation of protocol.
Treatment regimen	1. Anistreplase 30 U over 2-5 min IV and streptokinase placebo. 2. Placebo and Streptokinase 1.5 million U over 60 min.

TEAM-2

The Second Thrombolytic Trial of Eminase in Acute Myocardial Infarction

(continued)

Additional therapy	Heparin 5000-10,000 U bolus at the start of catheterization. IV infusion 1000 U/h was commenced after the angiography for >24 h. Diphenhydramine 25-50 mg IV was recommended.
Results	Early (mean 140 min) patency rate (TIMI flow 2-3) was 72% with APSAC and 73% with streptokinase. However, TIMI flow 3 was seen in 83% and 72%, respectively (p=0.03). Mean residual coronary artery stenosis was 74% vs 77.2%, respectively (p=0.02), in those who achieved TIMI flow 2-3. Reocclusion risk within 1-2 days was found in 1.0% and 2.1% of the APSAC and streptokinase patients. Enzymatic and electrocardiographic evolution was similar. In-hospital mortality was 5.9% vs 7.1% (p=0.61). Bleeding complications, stroke , allergic reactions, and cardiovascular com plications were similar.
Conclusions	Streptokinase and APSAC were equally effective and safe as thrombolytic therapy within 4 h of onset of acute myocardial infarction.

TAMI-5

Thrombolysis and Angioplasty in Myocardial Infarction- 5

Title	Evaluation of combination thrombolytic therapy and timing of cardiac catheterization in acute myocardial infarction. Results of Thrombolysis and Angioplasty in Myocardial Infarction- phase 5 randomized trial.
Authors	Califf RM, Topol EJ, Stack RS, et al.
Reference	Circulation 1991;83:1543-1556.
Disease	Acute myocardial infarction.
Purpose	To evaluate 3 thrombolytic regimens (tissue-type plasminogen activator (t-PA), urokinase, or both) and 2 strategies (immediate versus predischarge catheterization).
Design	Randomized, open label, 3X2 factorial, multicenter.
Patients	575 patients, age <76 years, with suspected acute myocardial infarction (chest pain ≤6 h; ST elevation ≥1 mm in ≥2 leads).
Follow-up	5-10 days (contrast ventriculogram and clinical evaluation).
Treatment regimen	1. Urokinase 1.5 million U bolus +1.5 million U infusion over 90 min. 2. t-PA 6 mg bolus, 54 mg over the first h, and 40 mg over 2 h. 3. Urokinase 1.5 million U over 60 min with 1mg/kg t-PA over 60 min (10% given as a bolus, maximal dose 90 mg). The early invasive strategy consisted of coronary angiography after 90 min of initiation of therapy with rescue angioplasty when indicated. The deferred strategy required coronary angiography 5-10 days after admission.

TAMI-5

Thrombolysis and Angioplasty in Myocardial Infarction- 5

(continued)

Additional therapy | Aspirin 325 mg/d. Heparin was started at the end of thrombolytic infusion at a dose of 1000 U/h for >48 h. In the aggressive strategy additional 5000 U heparin was given. Additional heparin was given during rescue angioplasty. Prophylactic lidocaine was used in most patients. Diltiazem 30-60 mg X3/d.

Results | Early patency rates were greater with the combination regimen (76%) versus 62% and 71% in the urokinase and t-PA arms (p=0.14). However, predischarge patency rates were similar. 5-10 days left ventricular ejection fraction was comparable among the three regimens and between the two strategies. Combination thrombolytic therapy was associated with less complicated clinical course and lower rate of reocclusion (2%) versus 7% and 11%, in the urokinase and t-PA regimens (p=0.04), and a lower rate of recurrent ischemia (25% versus 35% and 31%, respectively). Combination therapy was associated with the lower rates of the combined end point of death, stroke, reinfarction, reocclusion, heart failure, or recurrent ischemia (32% versus 45% and 40% for urokinase, and t-PA, respectively, p=0.04). Bleeding complications were comparable among the groups. Predischarge patency rates were 94% and 90% in the early invasive and early conservative strategies (p=0.065). Regional wall motion in the infarct zone was improved more with the early aggressive approach (-2.16 SDs/chord versus -2.49 SDs/chord, p=0.004). More patients in the early invasive strategy were free from adverse outcomes (67% versus 55%, p=0.004).

Conclusions | Combination thrombolytic therapy is more effective than single agent therapy for achievement of early and sustained reperfusion and for reducing the incidence of in-hospital complications. The early intervention strategy may result in better clinical outcome.

TAMI-7

Thrombolysis and Angioplasty in Myocardial Infarction VII

Title	Accelerated plasminogen activator dose regimens for coronary thrombolysis.
Authors	Wall TC, Califf RM, George BS, et al.
Reference	J Am Coll Cardiol 1992;19:482-489.
Disease	Acute myocardial infarction.
Purpose	To evaluate the efficacy of 5 different regimens of tissue plasminogen activator (t-PA) administration in acute myocardial infarction.
Design	Randomized, multicenter.
Patients	219 patients, >18 and <76 years old, with suspected acute myocardial infarction (>30 min pain unresponsive to sublingual nitrate, ≤6 h from onset of symptoms, ≥1 mm ST elevation in ≥2 leads or ST depression in V1-V4.
Follow-up	In-hospital events, pre-treatment and 5-10 days coronary angiography.
Treatment regimen	1. t-PA 1mg/kg over 30min (10% bolus), 0.25mg/kg over 30min. Max. dose 120mg. 2. t-PA 1.25mg/kg over 90min (20 mg bolus). Max. dose 120mg. 3. t-PA 0.75mg/kg over 30min (10% bolus), 0.50mg/kg over 60min. Max. dose 120mg. 4. t-PA 20mg bolus, 30min wait, 80mg over 120min. Max. dose 100mg. 5. t-PA 1mg/kg over 30min + urokinase 1.5 million U over 1h. Max. dose 90mg.

Additional therapy	Standard care including lidocaine, oxygen, morphine, and nitrates. Aspirin 325 mg/d. Heparin infusion 1,000 U/h started at the end of thrombolytic infusion and continued for 5-10 days. Metoprolol IV 15 mg if no contraindication existed.
Results	90 min patency rates were 63%, 61%, 83%, 67%, and 72% for protocols 1-5, respectively. Reocclusion occurred in 11%, 3%, 4%, 14%, and 3%, respectively. Protocol 3 achieved the highest rate of reperfusion and a low rate of reocclusion. Predischarge left ventricular ejection fraction was not statistically different among the groups. There was no difference in bleeding complications among the groups. Death, reocclusion, restenosis, and reinfarction tended to be less frequent in protocol 3, however, without statistical significance.
Conclusions	Accelerated t-PA administration according to protocol 3 is a relatively safe strategy achieving high 90 min patency rate and low reocclusion and complication rates.

ISIS-3

International Study of Infarct Survival 3

Title	ISIS-3: a randomized comparison of streptokinase vs tissue plasminogen activator vs anistreplase and of aspirin plus heparin vs aspirin alone among 41299 cases of suspected acute myocardial infarction.
Authors	ISIS-3 Collaborative Group.
Reference	Lancet 1992;339:753-770.
Disease	Acute myocardial infarction
Purpose	1. To compare three thrombolytic agents: tissue plasminogen activator (t-PA), streptokinase, and anisoylated plasminogen streptokinase activator complex (APSAC). 2. To compare treatment with heparin + aspirin with aspirin.
Design	Randomized, double blind (for thrombolytic agents) and open label (for heparin), 3X2 factorial, multicenter.
Patients	41,299 patients with suspected acute myocardial infarction within 24 h of onset of symptoms. No ECG criteria were used.
Follow-up	6 months.
Treatment regimen	1. Streptokinase 1.5 million U over 1 h. 2. t-PA 0.04 MU/kg as a bolus, and 0.36 MU/kg over 1 h, and then 0.067 MU/kg/h for 3 h. 3. APSAC 30 U over 3 min. Half of the patients received heparin subcutaneous 12,500 U X2/d for 1 week started 4h after initiation of thrombolytic therapy.
Additional therapy	162 mg chewed aspirin on admission and then 162 mg/d.

ISIS-3

International Study of Infarct Survival 3

(continued)

Results

Addition of heparin SC to aspirin resulted in excess of major non-cerebral hemorrhages (1.0% vs 0.8%, p<0.01) and of cerebral hemorrhages (0.56% vs 0.40%, p<0.05). However, total stroke occurred equally (1.28% vs 1.18%). Recurrent infarction occurred less in the heparin treated patients (3.16% vs 3.47%, p=0.09), especially during the scheduled heparin treatment. During the scheduled heparin treatment (0-7 days) mortality was 7.4% and 7.9% in the heparin and no heparin groups (p=0.06). However, 35-day and 6 months mortality were comparable.
APSAC was associated with more allergic reaction and non-cerebral bleeding and a trend towards more strokes than streptokinase. Reinfarction and 35-day mortality were comparable (3.47% and 10.6% vs 3.55% and 10.5% in the streptokinase and APSAC groups, respectively). There was no difference in 6-month survival between the groups. t-PA was associated with less allergic reactions than streptokinase, but with higher rates of non-cerebral bleeding. Stroke occurred in 1.04% of the streptokinase and 1.39% of the t-PA groups (p<0.01). t-PA was associated with less reinfarction (2.93% vs 3.47% in the t-PA and streptokinase groups, p<0.02) However, 35-day mortality was comparable (10.3% vs 10.6%, respectively). 6-month survival was similar.

Conclusions

It might be that heparin may produce at least a small improvement in survival and will reduce reinfarction, especially during the treatment period. There was no advantage of APSAC over streptokinase. The excess strokes observed with t-PA overshadows the reduction in reinfarction rate. t-PA is not better than streptokinase.

LATE

Late Assessment of Thrombolytic Efficacy

Title	Late assessment of thrombolytic efficacy (LATE) study with alteplase 6-24 hours after onset of acute myocardial infarction.
Authors	Late Study Group.
Reference	Lancet 1993;342:759-766.
Disease	Acute myocardial infarction.
Purpose	To assess the efficacy of intravenous thrombolytic therapy beginning more than 6 hours after the onset of symptoms.
Design	Randomized double-blind, placebo controlled, multicenter.
Patients	5711 patients with acute myocardial infarction >18 years old, 6-24 hours from onset of symptoms.
Follow-up	Clinical follow-up for 6 months (73% were followed up for 1 year).
Treatment regimen	Intravenous alteplase (r-tPA) 10 mg bolus, 50 mg infusion over 1 hour, and 20 mg/hour for two hours or matching placebo.
Additional therapy	Aspirin 75-360 mg/d. IV heparin for 48 hours was recommended.

LATE

Late Assessment of Thrombolytic Efficacy

(continued)

Results	35-day mortality for patients treated 6-12 hours after onset of symptoms was 8.9% versus 12.0% in the alteplase and placebo groups, respectively (95% CI 6.3-45.0%, p=0.02) 35-day mortality for patients treated >12 hours after onset of symptoms was 8.7% versus 9.2% in the alteplase and placebo groups, respectively (p=0.14).
Conclusions	Thrombolytic therapy reduces 35-day mortality even if given up to 12 hours after onset of symptoms.

EMERAS

Estudio Multicèntrico Estreptoquinasa Reùblicas de Amèrica del Sur

Title	Randomized trial of late thrombolysis in patients with suspected acute myocardial infarction.
Authors	EMERAS Collaborative Group.
Reference	Lancet 1993;342:767-772.
Disease	Acute myocardial infarction.
Purpose	To evaluate the efficacy of late treatment (6-24 h) with intravenous streptokinase for acute myocardial infarction.
Design	Randomized, double blind, placebo control, multicenter.
Patients	4534 patients with acute myocardial infarction > 6h and ≤ 24 h of onset of symptoms. ECG criteria were not required.
Follow-up	1 year.
Treatment regimen	Streptokinase 1.5 million U or placebo infused over 1 h.
Additional therapy	Aspirin 160 mg/d.

EMERAS

Estudio Multicèntrico Estreptoquinasa Reùblicas de Amèrica del Sur

(continued)

Results Side effects such as hypotension, allergic reactions and bleeding were more common with streptokinase therapy. There was no difference in in-hospital mortality between the streptokinase (11.9%) and placebo (12.4%) groups. Among the 2080 patients presenting 7-12 h from onset of symptoms there was a non significant trend towards less mortality with streptokinase (11.7% vs. 13.2%), whereas the mortality difference among the 1791 patients presenting 13-24 h after onset of symptoms was small (11.4% vs 10.7%). One year mortality was comparable between the streptokinase and placebo group.

Conclusions Streptokinase therapy 7-24 h after onset of symptoms did not show clear benefit. A modest reduction in mortality among patients treated 6-12 h after onset of symptoms is possible.

GUSTO-1

Global Utilization of Streptokinase and Tissue Plasminogen Activator for Occluded Coronary Arteries

Title	An international randomized trial comparing four thrombolytic strategies for acute myocardial infarction.
Authors	The GUSTO Investigators.
Reference	N Engl J Med 1993;329:673-682.
Disease	Acute myocardial infarction.
Purpose	To compare the effects of four thrombolytic strategies on outcome.
Design	Randomized, open label, multicenter.
Patients	41,021 patients with acute myocardial infarction < 6 hours from onset of symptoms with chest pain>20 min and ST segment elevation ≥0.1 mV in ≥2 limb leads , or ≥0.2 mV in ≥2 precordial leads.
Follow-up	30 days clinical follow-up.
Treatment regimen	1. intravenous streptokinase 1.5 million U over 60 min with subcutaneous heparin 12,500 U BID; 2. streptokinase 1.5 million U over 60 min with intravenous heparin (5000 U bolus and 1000U/hour); 3. accelerated t-PA (15 mg bolus, 0.75 mg/kg over 30 min, and 0.5 mg/kg over 60 min) with intravenous heparin (5000 U bolus and 1000U/hour); and 4. the combination of intravenous t-PA (1.0 mg/kg over 60 min, with 10% given as a bolus) and streptokinase (1.0 million U over 60 min) with intravenous heparin (5000 U bolus and 1000U/hour).
Additional therapy	Chewable aspirin 160 mg on admission and 160-325 mg/d thereafter. IV 5 mg atenolol in two divided doses, followed by 50-100 mg/d PO was recommended if no contraindications existed.

GUSTO-1

Global Utilization of Streptokinase and Tissue Plasminogen Activator for Occluded Coronary Arteries

(continued)

Results

30-day mortality was 7.2% for the streptokinase with SC heparin group; 7.4% for the streptokinase and IV heparin group, 6.3% for the accelerated t-PA and IV heparin group; and 7.0% for the combination group. Thus, 14% reduction (95% CI 5.9-21.3%) in 30-day mortality for accelerated t-PA as compared with the two groups of streptokinase therapy. Hemorrhagic stroke occurred in 0.49%, 0.54%, 0.72%, and 0.94% in the four groups, respectively ($p=0.03$ for the difference between t-PA and streptokinase; $p<0.001$ for the combination therapy compared to streptokinase-only). A combined end point of death or disabling stroke was lower in the t-PA treated patients (6.9%) than in patients receiving the streptokinase-only regimens (7.8%) ($p=0.006$).

Conclusions

The mortality of patients with acute myocardial infarction treated with accelerated t-PA and intravenous heparin is lower than those receiving streptokinase with either subcutaneous or intravenous heparin.

GUSTO-1 (angiographic substudy)

Global Utilization of Streptokinase and Tissue Plasminogen Activator for Occluded Coronary Arteries

---

Title	The effects of tissue plasminogen activator, streptokinase, or both on coronary-artery patency, ventricular function, and survival after acute myocardial infarction.
Authors	The GUSTO Angiographic Investigators.
Reference	N Engl J Med 1993;329:1615-1622.
Disease	Acute myocardial infarction.
Purpose	To compare the speed of reperfusion and the effect on left ventricular function and outcome of tissue plasminogen activator and streptokinase.
Design	Randomized, open label, multicenter.
Patients	2431 patients with acute myocardial infarction < 6 hours from onset of symptoms with chest pain>20 min and ST segment elevation ≥0.1 mV in ≥2 limb leads , or ≥0.2 mV in ≥2 precordial leads.
Follow-up	Patients were randomized to cardiac catheterization at 90 min, 180 min, 24 h or 5-7 days. The group that underwent coronary angiography at 90 min underwent it again after 5-7 days. 30 days clinical follow-up.
Treatment regimen	1. intravenous streptokinase 1.5 million U over 60 min with subcutaneous heparin 12,500 U BID; 2. streptokinase 1.5 million U over 60 min with intravenous heparin (5000 U bolus and 1000 U/hour); 3. accelerated t-PA (15 mg bolus, 0.75 mg/kg over 30 min, and 0.5 mg/kg over 60 min) with intravenous heparin (5000 U bolus and 1000 U/hour); and 4. the combination of intravenous t-PA (1.0 mg/kg over 60 min, with 10% given as a bolus) and streptokinase (1.0 million U over 60 min) with intravenous heparin (5000 U bolus and 1000 U/hour).

GUSTO-1 (angiographic substudy)

Global Utilization of Streptokinase and Tissue Plasminogen Activator for Occluded Coronary Arteries

(continued)

Additional therapy

Chewable aspirin 160 mg on admission and 160-325 mg/d thereafter. IV 5 mg atenolol in two divided doses, followed by 50-100 mg/d PO was recommended if no contraindications existed.

Results

90 min patency rate was 54% in the streptokinase + heparin SC, 60% in the streptokinase+ heparin IV, 81% in the t-PA, and 73% in the combination therapy (p<0.001 for t-PA vs the 2 streptokinase groups). However, at 180 min the difference disappeared. TIMI flow III at 90 min was achieved by 29%, 32%, 54%, and 38%, respectively (p<0.001 for t-PA vs the 2 streptokinase groups). There was no significant differences among the groups in the rate of reocclusion. Regional wall motion was better in the t-PA than the other 3 groups. 30-day mortality was 6.5%, 7.5%, 5.3%, and 7.8%, respectively. Mortality was correlated with lack of patency at 90 min (8.9% in patients with TIMI flow grade 0-1 at 90 min vs 4.4% in patients with TIMI flow grade 3, p=0.009).

Conclusions

Accelerated t-PA regimen achieved faster and more complete reperfusion and was associated with better regional wall motion and outcome.

Update

A one year follow-up study [Califf RM, et al. circ. 1996;94:1233-1238] showed that one year mortality rates remained in favor of t-PA (9.1%) versus streptokinase with subcutaneous heparin (10.1%, p=0.01), versus steptokinase with IV heparin (10.1%, p=.009). Combination of IV t-PA and streptokinase had an intermediate outcome (9.9%).

EMIP

The European Myocardial Infarction Project Group

Authors	The European Myocardial Infarction Project Group
Title	Prehospital thrombolytic therapy in patients with suspected acute myocardial infarction.
Reference	N Engl J Med 1993;329:383-389.
Disease	Acute myocardial infarction.
Purpose	To compare the efficacy and safety of pre-hospital versus in-hospital administration of thrombolytic therapy for patients with suspected acute myocardial infarction.
Study Design	Randomized, double blind, multicenter.
Follow-up	30 day clinical follow-up.
Treatment regimen	Patients were randomized to 30 units of anistreplase IV over 4-5 min given by the emergency medical personnel outside the hospital, followed by placebo after hospitalization, or to placebo outside the hospital followed by 30 units of anistreplase after admission.
Concomitant therapy	No limitations, except for anticoagulant therapy.
Patients	5469 patients with chest pain of ≥30 min, or pain unresponsive to nitrates, ≤6 h of onset of symptoms. Patients on oral anticoagulants, with a history of stroke, major trauma, or bleeding diathesis were excluded. Patients were stratified according to the presence of ST segment elevation on the qualifying ECG.

EMIP

The European Myocardial Infarction Project Group

(continued)

Results The patients in the pre-hospital therapy group received thrombolytic therapy 55 min earlier than those in the hospital therapy group. 30 day mortality was 9.7% vs 11.1% in the pre-hospital and hospital groups (risk reduction 13%, 95% CI -1 to 26%, p=0.08). Cardiac mortality was 8.3% vs 9.8%, respectively (risk reduction 16%, 95% CI 0 to 29%, p=0.049). There was no obvious correlation between the reduction in 30 day mortality and the time interval between the onset of symptoms and the first injection. During the preadmission period there were more patients with ventricular fibrillation (2.5% vs 1.6%, p=0.02), shock (6.3% vs 3.9%, p<0.001), and stroke (0.1% vs 0, p=0.09) in the pre-hospital therapy than the in-hospital group. However, there was no differences between the groups in the incidence of bleeding, the overall incidence of stroke, ventricular fibrillation, and shock during the hospital period.

Conclusions Pre-hospital administration of thrombolytic therapy for patients with suspected acute myocardial infarction is feasible and safe. Although overall mortality was not reduced, cardiac mortality was significantly reduced.

MITI-2

The Myocardial Infarction Triage and Intervention Trial

Authors	Weaver DW, Cerqueira M, Hallstrom AP, et al.
Title	Prehospital-initiated vs hospital-initiated thrombolytic therapy. The myocardial infarction triage and intervention trial.
Reference	JAMA 1993;270:1211-1216.
Disease	Acute myocardial infarction.
Purpose	To evaluate the effect of pre-hospital vs in-hospital administration of thrombolytic therapy for suspected acute myocardial infarction.
Study Design	Randomized, controlled, multicenter.
Follow-up	In-hospital clinical events. Estimation of final infarct size by thallium single photon emission tomography and left ventricular function by radionuclide ventriculography at 30 days.
Treatment regimen	Patients were randomized to either pre-hospital or in-hospital initiation of IV aspirin 325 mg and alteplase 100 mg infusion over 3 h. No placebo was given in the field to the hospital treated group.
Concomitant therapy	Standard care: oxygen, morphine, lidocaine, atropine, vasopressors or diuretics when indicated. IV heparin 5000 U bolus followed by continuous infusion for ≥48 h was started upon admission.
Patients	360 patients, ≤75 years old, with suspected acute myocardial infarction, within 6 h of onset of symptoms. Patients with risk factors for bleeding were excluded.

MITI-2

The Myocardial Infarction Triage and Intervention Trial

(continued)

Results

98% of the patients had subsequent evidence of acute myocardial infarction. Initiation of therapy before admission shortened the time interval from onset of symptoms to therapy from 110 to 77 min (p<0.001). 23% of the prehospital group vs 7% of the in-hospital group had resolution of pain upon admission (p<0.001). However there was no difference between the groups in the composite score of death, stroke, serious bleeding, and infarct size (406.4 vs 400.4 for the pre-hospital vs in-hospital groups, p=0.64), total mortality (5.7% vs 8.1%, p=0.49), infarct size (6.1% vs 6.5%, p=0.72), or ejection fraction (53% vs 54%, p=0.34). A secondary analysis of the time to therapy and outcome demonstrated that treatment initiated within 70 min of onset of symptoms was associated with better outcome (composite score, p=0.009; mortality 1.2% vs 8.7%, p=0.04; infarct size 4.9% vs 11.2%, p<0.001; and ejection fraction 53% vs 49%, p=0.03) than later treatment. Identification of patients eligible for thrombolytic therapy by paramedics reduced the time interval from hospitalization to therapy from 60 min (for non-randomized patients) to 20 min (in the in-hospital therapy allocated group).

Conclusions

There was no improvement in outcome associated with pre-hospital administration of thrombolytic therapy. However, treatment within 70 min of onset of symptoms was associated with better outcome. Prehospital identification of patients eligible for thrombolytic therapy was associated with shortening of the time interval to therapy.

TIMI-4

Thrombolysis in Myocardial Infarction 4 Trial

Title	Comparison of front-loaded recombinant tissue-type plasminogen activator, anistreplase and combination thrombolytic therapy for acute myocardial infarction: Results of the Thrombolysis in Myocardial Infarction (TIMI) 4 trial.
Authors	Cannon CP, McCabe CH, Diver DJ, et al.
Reference	J Am Coll Cardiol 1994;24:1602-1610.
Disease	Acute myocardial infarction.
Purpose	To compare three regimens of thrombolytic therapy: anistreplase (APSAC), front-loaded recombinant tissue-type plasminogen activator (rt-PA) or combination of the two agents.
Design	Randomized, double blind, multicenter study.
Patients	382 patients with acute myocardial infarction <80 years old < 6 hours from onset of symptoms with chest pain>30 min and ST segment elevation ≥0.1 mV in ≥2 contiguous leads or with new left bundle branch block.
Follow-up	90 min and 18-36 h coronary angiography. Predischarge technetium-99m sestamibi scan. 6 week and 1 year follow-up.
Treatment regimen	Front-loaded rt-PA; APSAC (Eminase); or a combination of rt-PA and APSAC.
Additional therapy	Heparin (5000 U bolus and infusion) and aspirin 325 mg/d Intravenous and oral metoprolol.

TIMI-4

Thrombolysis in Myocardial Infarction 4 Trial

(continued)

Results

At 90 min, the incidence of TIMI grade 3 flow was 60.2%, 42.9%, and 44.8% of the rt-PA, APSAC, and combination-treated patients (rt-PA vs. APSAC, p<0.01; rt-PA vs. combination, p=0.02). The incidence of unsatisfactory outcome (death, severe heart failure, LVEF<40%, reinfarction, TIMI grade flow<2 at 90 min or 18-36 h, reocclusion, major hemorrhage, or severe anaphylaxis) was 41.3%, 49%, and 53.6% for the rt-PA, APSAC, and combination therapy (rt-PA vs. APSAC, p=0.19; rt-PA vs. combination, p=0.06). Six week mortality was 2.2%, 8.8%, and 7.2%, respectively (rt-PA vs. APSAC, p=0.02; rt-PA vs. combination, p=0.06).

Conclusions

Front-loaded rt-PA is associated with higher rates of early reperfusion and trends toward better clinical outcome and survival than either APSAC or a combination of rt-PA and APSAC.

INJECT

International Joint Efficacy Comparison of Thrombolytics

Title	Randomized, double-blind comparison of reteplase double-bolus administration with streptokinase in acute myocardial infarction (INJECT): trial to investigate equivalence.
Authors	International Joint Efficacy Comparison of Thrombolytics.
Reference	Lancet 1995;346:329-336.
Disease	Acute myocardial infarction.
Purpose	To compare the effect of reteplase and streptokinase in acute myocardial infarction.
Design	Randomized, double blind, multicenter.
Patients	6010 patients, ≥18 year old, with chest pain of ≥30 min, within 12 h of onset of symptoms, ST elevation ≥1 mm in ≥2 limb leads, or ≥2 mm in ≥2 precordial leads, or bundle branch block.
Follow-up	6 months clinical follow-up.
Treatment regimen	Two boluses of 10 MU reteplase given 30 min apart +1 h infusion of placebo streptokinase, or 2 retaplase placebo boluses and 1.5 MU IV streptokinase.
Additional therapy	Aspirin 250-320 mg initially, then 75-150 mg/d. IV heparin 5000 U before infusion of thrombolytics, and heparin infusion 1000 U/h 60 min after trial infusion for >24 h.

INJECT

International Joint Efficacy Comparison of Thrombolytics

(continued)

Results 35 day mortality was 9.02% vs 9.53% in the reteplase and streptokinase groups (a difference of -0.51%, 95% CI -1.98% to 0.96%). 6 month mortality was 11.02% vs 12.05%, respectively (a difference of -1.03%, 95% CI -2.65% to 0.59%, p=0.217). There was a non-significant excess of in-hospital strokes in the reteplase patients (1.23% vs 1.00%). Bleeding events were similar (total: 15.0% vs 15.3%, requiring transfusion: 0.7% vs 1.0%, respectively). Hypotension during hospitalization was more common with streptokinase (17.6% vs 15.5%, p<0.05). Allergic reactions occurred more often with streptokinase (1.8% vs 1.1%, p<0.05).

Conclusions Reteplase is a safe and an effective thrombolytic agent.

RAPID

Reteplase versus Alteplase Infusion in Acute Myocardial Infarction

Title	More rapid, complete, and stable coronary thrombolysis with bolus administration of reteplase compared with alteplase infusion in acute myocardial infarction.
Authors	Smalling RW, Bode C, Kalbfleisch J, et al.
Reference	Circulation 1995;91:2725-2732.
Disease	Acute myocardial infarction.
Purpose	To compare the 90 min coronary patency rates of bolus administration of reteplase (r-PA) and standard-dose alteplase (tPA).
Design	Randomized, open label, multicenter.
Patients	606 patients, age 18-75 years, with ≥30 min chest pain and ST elevation of ≥1 mm in the limb leads and ≥2 mm in the precordial leads, within 6 h of onset of symptoms. Patients with left bundle branch block, prior coronary artery bypass surgery, previous Q wave infarction in the same territory, previous angioplasty within 2 weeks, previous cerebral vascular event, or severe hypertension were excluded.
Follow-up	30 min, 60 min, 90 min and 5-14 days coronary angiography.
Treatment regimen	1. 15 MU r-PA as a single bolus. 2. 10 MU r-PA bolus followed by 5 MU 30 min later. 3. 10 MU r-PA bolus followed by 10 MU 30 min later. 4. TPA 60 mg over 1 h (6-10 mg as an initial bolus) followed by 40 mg over 2 h.
Additional therapy	Soluble aspirin 200-325 mg/d. IV heparin 5000 U bolus before thrombolytic therapy, followed by 1000 U/h for ≥24 h.

RAPID

Reteplase versus Alteplase Infusion in Acute Myocardial Infarction

(continued)

Results

60 min patency (TIMI flow grade II and III) were 67.0%, 72.1%, 77.6%, and 66.3% in groups 1-4 (r-PA 10+10 vs TPA p=0.079). At 90 min, patency rates were 62.8%, 66.7%, 85.2%, and 77.2%, respectively (r-PA 10+10 vs TPA p=0.084). Late patency was 85.5%, 80.5%, 95.1%, and 87.8% (r-PA 10+10 vs TPA p=0.04). TIMI flow III was higher in the r-PA 10+10 than TPA at 60 min (51.0% vs 32.7%, p=0.009), at 90 min (62.7% vs 49.0%, p=0.019), and at discharge (87.8% vs 70.7%, p<0.001). Global left ventricular function at 90 min was similar in the TPA and r-PA 10+10 groups. However, at discharge ejection fraction was higher in the r-PA 10+10 (53±1.3% vs 49±1.3%, p=0.034). Regional wall motion improved in the r-PA 10+10 from 90 min to predischarge, while in the TPA group there was no improvement. There was a trend towards less rescue angioplasty in the r-PA 10+10 than TPA group (p=0.11). The need for blood transfusion was similar (4.5% in the TPA vs 3.9% in the r-PA 10+10), while intracranial bleeding occurred in 2.6% vs 0%, respectively. Reocclusion occurred in 7.8% of the TPA vs 2.9% in the r-PA 10+10 (p=NS). The 30-day mortality was 3.9% vs 1.9%, respectively. Reinfarction rate and the incidence of heart failure were similar between the groups.

Conclusions

r-PA given as a double bolus of 10 MU+ 10 MU 30 min apart resulted in more rapid and complete reperfusion than standard-dose TPA and was associated with improved global and regional left ventricular function at discharge.

RAPID II

Reteplase versus Alteplase Infusion in Acute Myocardial Infarction II

Title	Randomized comparison of coronary thrombolysis achieved with double-bolus reteplase (recombinant plasminogen activator) and front-loaded, accelerated alteplase (recombinant tissue plasminogen activator) in patients with acute myocardial infarction
Authors	Bode C, Smalling RW, Berg G, et al.
Reference	Circulation 1996;94:891-898.
Disease	Acute myocardial infarction.
Purpose	To assess whether a double-bolus regimen of reteplase, a deletion mutant of wild-type tissue plasminogen activator, results in better 90-minute coronary artery patency rates compared with accelerated front-loaded infusion of alteplase (tissue plasminogen activator).
Design	Randomized, open-label, parallel-group, multicenter.
Patients	324 patients, $>$18 years old with $\geq$30 min of chest pain that was not relieved by nitroglycerin, $\leq$12 h from onset of pain, and ST segment elevation of $\geq$0.1 mV in limb leads or $\geq$0.2 mV in precordial leads, or left bundle branch block. Patients with prior coronary artery bypass surgery, previous stroke or known intracranial structural abnormalities, PTCA within 2 weeks, previous Q wave myocardial infarction in the same territory, severe hypertension, use of oral anticoagulants, recent ($<$3 months) major surgery or active or potential internal bleeding were excluded.
Follow-up	Coronary angiography at 30, 60, 90 min, and 5-14 days after initiation of therapy, clinical follow-up for 35 days.

RAPID II

Reteplase versus Alteplase Infusion in Acute Myocardial Infarction II

(continued)

Treatment regimen Randomization to a bolus of reteplase (10 MU given over 2-3 min) at the start of therapy and after 30 min, or to alteplase (15 mg bolus, 0.75 mg/kg over 30 min (maximum 50 mg), 0.5 mg/kg over 60 min (maximum 35 mg).

Additional therapy Aspirin 160 to 350 mg/d. Intravenous heparin, 5000 IU bolus followed by 1000 IU/h for ≥24 h. Target aPTT 2.0 times the control value.

Results 90 min following initiation of therapy, infarct related coronary artery patency (TIMI flow grade 2 or 3) was higher in the reteplase group (83.4% vs 73.3%, p=0.031). TIMI flow grade 3 was achieved in 59.9% vs 45.2%, respectively (p=0.011). At 60 min, TIMI flow grade 2 or 3 was found in 81.8% of the reteplase group vs 66.1% in the alteplase group (p=0.032), and TIMI flow grade 3 was found in 51.2% vs 37.4%, respectively (p=0.006). Follow-up angiograms were available in 75.7% and 72.9% of the reteplase and alteplase-treated patients. Late overall and TIMI flow grade 3 patency were comparable between the groups. Patients treated with reteplase had better patency in all time-to-treatment categories. Additional interventions to restore flow in the infarct related artery during the first 6 hours was lower in the reteplase group (13.6% vs 26.5%; p=0.004). The incidence of reocclusion during hospitalization was comparable (9.0% vs 7.0% for reteplase and alteplase, respectively, p=0.61). 35-day mortality was 4.1% vs 8.4%, respectively (p=0.11). The incidence of stroke (1.8% vs 2.6%) was similar. The composite end point of unsatisfactory outcome at 35 days (death, reinfarction, congestive heart failure or shock, or an ejection fraction of <40%) was comparable (21.3% vs 22.6% in the reteplase and alteplase groups). 12.4% vs 9.7% of the patients, respectively, required transfusion (p=0.43). There was no difference in global or infarct zone left ventricular function between the groups.

Conclusions Double bolus dose of reteplase was associated with higher rates of reperfusion at 60 and 90-min after initiation of therapy than front-loaded alteplase infusion, without an increase in the risk of complications.

1. Acute Myocardial Infarction
b. PTCA Versus Thrombolytic Therapy

PAMI-1

Primary Angioplasty in Myocardial Infarction 1

Title	a. A comparison of immediate angioplasty with thrombolytic therapy for acute myocardial infarction. b. Predictors of in-hospital and 6-month outcome after acute myocardial infarction in the reperfusion era: the primary angioplasty in myocardial infarction (PAMI) trial.
Authors	a. Grines CL, Browne KF, Marco J, et al. b. Stone GW, Grines CL, Browne KF, et al.
Reference	a. N Engl J Med 1993;328:673-679. b. J Am Coll Cardiol 1995;25:370-377.
Disease	Acute myocardial infarction.
Purpose	To compare the results of primary coronary angioplasty with intravenous tissue plasminogen activator for acute myocardial infarction.
Design	Randomized, open label, multicenter.
Patients	395 patients within 12 h of onset of chest pain with ≥1 mm ST elevation in ≥2 adjacent leads. No age limit.
Follow-up	a. Clinical follow-up at 6 months. Radionuclide ventriculography within 24 h and at 6 weeks. Exercise thallium scan predischarge. b. 6 month clinical follow-up.
Treatment regimen	1. Tissue plasminogen activator (t-PA) 100 mg over 3 h. 2. Immediate coronary angiography and angioplasty if suitable.

PAMI-1

Primary Angioplasty in Myocardial Infarction 1

(continued)

Additional therapy Intravenous nitroglycerin for ≥24 h, chewed aspirin 325 mg and 325 mg/d thereafter, and 10,000 U bolus heparin started before randomization. Intravenous heparin infusion was continued for 3-5 days. Diltiazem 30-60 mg X4/d.

Results a. 90% of the patients assigned to angioplasty underwent the procedure. The success rate was 97%. In-hospital mortality was 6.5% and 2.6% in the t-PA and angioplasty groups, respectively (p=0.06). Reinfarction or death occurred in 12.0% and 5.1%, respectively (p=0.02). Intracranial hemorrhage occurred in 2.0% and 0, respectively (p=0.05). The mean length of the hospital stay was shorter in the angioplasty group (7.5±3.3 vs. 8.4±4.6 days, p=0.03). The mean ejection fraction at rest and during exercise were similar at 6 weeks. By 6 months death in 7.9% and 3.7% (p=0.08), and recurrent infarction or death had occurred in 16.8% and 8.5% (p=0.02) of the t-PA and angioplasty groups, respectively.

b. By 6 months, cumulative mortality and reinfarction rate was 8.2% and 17.0% in the angioplasty and t-PA groups (p=0.02). By multiple logistic regression analysis only advanced age, prior heart failure, and treatment with t-PA vs angioplasty were independently associated with increased in-hospital mortality.

Conclusions Primary angioplasty resulted in lower occurrence of nonfatal recurrent infarction or death, and lower rates of intracranial hemorrhage than t-PA.

A Comparison of Immediate Coronary Angioplasty with Intravenous Streptokinase in Acute Myocardial Infarction.

Title	A comparison of immediate coronary angioplasty with intravenous streptokinase in acute myocardial infarction.
Authors	Zijlstra F, de Boer MJ, Hoorntje JCA. et al.
Reference	N Engl J Med 1993;328:680-684.
Disease	Acute myocardial infarction.
Purpose	To compare the results of immediate coronary angioplasty with intravenous streptokinase infusion for acute myocardial infarction.
Design	Randomized, open labeled, one center.
Patients	142 patients, age <76 years, with acute myocardial infarction (symptoms ≥ 30 min; < 6 h from onset of symptoms, or 6-24 h if there was evidence of continuing ischemia; ST elevation >1 mm in ≥2 leads).
Follow-up	In-hospital recurrent ischemia, predischarge symptom-limited exercise test, radionuclide ventriculography, and coronary angiography.
Treatment regimen	1. Streptokinase 1.5 million U over 1 h. 2. Immediate coronary angiography and angioplasty.
Additional therapy	Aspirin 300 mg IV, and then 300 mg/d orally. Intravenous nitroglycerin and intravenous heparin for >48 h.

A Comparison of Immediate Coronary Angioplasty with Intravenous Streptokinase in Acute Myocardial Infarction.

(continued)

Results

Death occurred in 4 (6%) of the 72 patients that received streptokinase, but in none of the 70 patients assigned to angioplasty (p=0.13). Recurrent infarction occurred in 9 (13%) patients that received streptokinase, but in none of the patients assigned to angioplasty (p=0.003). Post infarction angina developed in 14 (19%) and 4 (6%) patients in the streptokinase and angioplasty groups (p=0.02). Mean left ventricular ejection fraction before discharge was 45±12% in the streptokinase group, and 51±11% in the angioplasty group (p=0.004). The infarct related artery was patent in 68% and 91%, respectively (p=0.001). Residual stenosis was 76±19% and 36±20%, respectively (p<0.001). There was no difference in the complication rate between the groups. Ischemic ST segment depression during exercise test developed in 41% and 21% of the streptokinase and angioplasty groups (p=0.01). Left ventricular ejection fraction during exercise was 46±15% and 52±14%, respectively (p=0.02).

Conclusions

Immediate angioplasty was associated with higher rates of patency, lower grade of residual stenosis, better left ventricular function, and less recurrent ischemia and infarction than intravenous streptokinase therapy.

Immediate Angioplasty Compared With the Administration of a Thrombolytic Agent.

Title	Immediate angioplasty compared with the administration of a thrombolytic agent followed by conservative treatment for myocardial infarction.
Authors	Gibbons AJ, Holmes DR, Reeder GS, et al.
Reference	N Engl J Med 1993;328:685-691.
Disease	Acute myocardial infarction.
Purpose	To compare direct angioplasty with administration of thrombolytic agent followed by conservative approach in the management of acute myocardial infarction.
Design	Randomized, open labeled, one center.
Patients	103 patients, age <80 years, with acute myocardial infarction (pain ≥30 min, ≤12 h from onset of symptoms, ST elevation of ≥1 mm in ≥2 adjacent leads, or new ST depression of ≥2 mm in ≥2 precordial leads. Patients with contraindication to thrombolytic therapy or in cardiogenic shock were excluded.
Follow-up	Technetium 99m sestamibi scan before therapy, and 6-14 days later. radionuclide ventriculography at rest predischarge and at 6 weeks.
Treatment regimen	1. Double chain tissue plasminogen activator (duteplase) 0.6 million U/kg over 4 h. Heparin 5000 U bolus and infusion for 5 days, and then subcutaneous 12,500 U X2/d. 2. Heparin 5,000 +10,000 U bolus, coronary angioplasty. Intravenous heparin infusion for 5 days.
Additional therapy	162.5 mg of chewable aspirin, and 162.5 mg/d thereafter. ß blockers if not contraindicated.

Results	56 patients received t-PA (time from onset of symptoms to start of infusion 232±174 min), and 47 underwent angioplasty (first balloon inflation 277±144 min after onset of symptoms). Mortality was similar (2 in each group). Myocardial salvage for anterior infarction, as assessed by the difference between the pre-treatment to predischarge MIBI defect size, was 27±21% and 31±21% of the left ventricle, in the t-PA and angioplasty groups, respectively. For non-anterior infarctions salvage was 7±13% and 5±10%, respectively. There was no difference in ejection fraction between the groups at discharge or after 6 weeks.
Conclusions	There was no difference in myocardial salvage between immediate angioplasty and intravenous thrombolytic therapy followed by conservative therapy.

1. Acute Myocardial Infarction
c. Anticoagulation

HART

Heparin-Aspirin Reperfusion Trial

Title	A comparison between heparin and low-dose aspirin as adjunctive therapy with tissue plasminogen activator for acute myocardial infarction.
Authors	Hsia J, Hamilton WP, Kleiman N, et al.
Reference	N Engl J Med 1990;323:1433-1437.
Disease	Acute myocardial infarction.
Purpose	To compare early intravenous heparin with oral aspirin as adjunctive therapy to tissue plasminogen activator for acute myocardial infarction.
Design	Randomized, open label, multicenter.
Patients	193 patients, age <76 years, with chest pain and ST elevation ≥ 1 mm in ≥ 2 contiguous leads, within 6 h from onset of symptoms.
Follow-up	7-24 h and 7 day cardiac catheterization. 7 day clinical course.
Treatment regimen	1. Oral aspirin 80 mg/d, started with the t-PA for 7 days. 2. IV heparin 5000 U bolus, followed by 1000 U/h, started with the t-PA for 7 days.
Additional therapy	Intravenous tissue plasminogen activator (t-PA) 6 mg bolus, 54 mg over the first h, 20 mg over the second h, and 20 mg over 4 h.

HART

Heparin-Aspirin Reperfusion Trial

(continued)

Results At the time of the first angiogram, 82% and 52% of the infarct related arteries of the patients assigned to heparin and aspirin were patent ($p<0.0001$). Of the arteries that were initially patent, 88% and 95% in the heparin and aspirin groups remained patent after 7.4±2.4 days ($p=0.17$). The number of bleeding events and recurrent ischemia were similar between the groups. The mortality rate was 1.9% vs 4.0% in the heparin and aspirin groups, respectively (p=NS).

Conclusions Coronary patency rate improved when heparin was added to t-PA compare to when aspirin was added.

TIMI-5

Thrombolysis in Myocardial Infarction 5 Trial

Title	A pilot trial of recombinant desulfatohirudin compared with heparin in conjunction with tissue-type plasminogen activator and aspirin for acute myocardial infarction: Results of the Thrombolysis in Myocardial Infarction (TIMI) 5 trial.
Authors	Cannon CP, McCabe CH, Henry TD, et al.
Reference	J Am Coll Cardiol 1994;23:993-1003.
Disease	Acute myocardial infarction.
Purpose	To compare the efficacy of recombinant desulfatohirudin (hirudin) to heparin as adjunctive therapy to thrombolysis in acute myocardial infarction.
Design	Randomized, multicenter, dose escalation trial.
Patients	246 patients with acute myocardial infarction < 6 hours from onset of symptoms with chest pain >30 min and ST segment elevation ≥0.1 mV in ≥2 contiguous leads or with new left bundle branch block.
Follow-up	90 min and 18-36 h coronary angiography. In-hospital clinical events.
Treatment regimen	intravenous heparin or hirudin at one of four escalating doses (Bolus (mg/kg) and intravenous infusion mg/kg per hour) of 0.15 and 0.05; 0.1 and 0.1; 0.3 and 0.1; and 0.6 and 0.2, respectively) for 5 days.
Additional therapy	front-loaded tissue-type plasminogen activator and aspirin 160 mg/d. Intravenous and oral metoprolol.

Results

The primary efficacy end point (achievement of TIMI 3 flow at 90 min and 18-36 h without death or reinfarction before the second angiography) was achieved in 61.8% and 49.4% of the hirudin and heparin- treated patients , respectively (p=0.07). While 90 min patency of the infarct related artery was similar, at 18-36 h, 97.8% and 89.2 % of the hirudin and heparin- treated patients had an open artery, respectively (p=0.01). In-hospital death or reinfarction occurred in 6.8% and 16.7% of the hirudin and heparin groups, respectively (p=0.02). Major hemorrhage occurred in 1.2% and 4.7% of the patients, respectively (p=0.09).

Conclusions

Hirudin is a relatively safe drug and has a several advantages over heparin, as an adjunctive to front-loaded tissue plasminogen activator therapy.

Title	Beneficial effects of RheothRx injection in patients receiving thrombolytic therapy for acute myocardial infarction. Results of a randomized, double-blind, placebo-controlled trial.
Authors	Schaer GL, Spaccavento LJ, Browne KF, et al.
Reference	Circulation 1996;94:298-307.
Disease	Acute myocardial infarction.
Purpose	To evaluate the safety and efficacy of adjunctive therapy with RheothRx (poloxamer 188, a surfactanct with hemorheological and antithrombotic properties) in patients with acute myocardial infarction undergoing thrombolytic therapy.
Design	Randomized, double blind, placebo-controlled, multicenter.
Patients	114 patients, ≥18 years old, with suspected acute myocardial infarction (chest pain ≥30 min, ST elevation in ≥2 leads. All patients received thrombolytic therapy within 6 h of onset of symptoms. Patients with serum creatinine ≥3.0 mg/dL were excluded.
Follow-up	Clinical follow-up and ^{99m}Tc sestamibi tomographic imaging with radionuclide ventriculography before reperfusion and 5-7 days after infarction.
Treatment regimen	RheothRx (150 or 300 mg/kg over 1 h and then 15 or 30 mg/kg/h for 47 h) or placebo infusion was initiated immediately after initiation of thrombolytic therapy.
Additional therapy	Thrombolytic therapy (tPA or streptokinase). Chewable aspirin, nitrates, IV followed by oral β-blocker and heparin for ≥48 h.

Results

75 patients were randomized to RheothRx and 39 to placebo. Baseline characteristics were not significantly different between the groups. RheothRx-treated patients had a 38% reduction in median infarct size (25th and 75th percentile) compared with placebo (16% (7,30) vs 26% (9,43); p=0.031), greater median myocardial salvage (13% (7,20) vs 4% (1,15); p=0.033), and higher ejection fraction (52% (43,60) vs 46% (35,60); p=0.02). RheothRx treated patients had lower rate of reinfarction (1% vs 13%, p=0.016). Therapy was well tolerated without adverse hemodynamic effects or bleeding.

Conclusions

Therapy with RheothRx was effective in reduction of infarct size and preservation of left ventricular function in patients undergoing thrombolytic therapy for acute myocardial infarction.

TIMI 9B

Thrombolysis and Thrombin Inhibition in Myocardial Infarction 9B

Title	Hirudin in acute myocardial infarction. Thrombolysis and thrombin inhibition in myocardial infarction (TIMI) 9B trial.
Authors	Antman EM, for the TIMI 9B Investigators.
Reference	Circulation 1996;94:911-921.
Disease	Acute myocardial infarction.
Purpose	To compare the efficacy and safety of recombinant desulfatohirudin (Hirudin) with heparin as adjunctive therapy to thrombolysis and aspirin in acute myocardial infarction.
Design	Randomized, double blind, multicenter.
Patients	3002 Patients, ≥21 years old, with acute myocardial infarction with ≥1 mm ST segment elevation in ≥2 leads or new LBBB, within 12 h of onset of symptoms, and no contraindications to thrombolytic therapy. Patients with serum creatinine >2.0 mg/dl, cardiogenic shock, or were receiving therapeutic doses of anticoagulants were excluded.
Follow-up	30 day clinical follow-up.
Treatment regimen	Randomization to heparin or hirudin. Therapy started within 60 min after thrombolysis and continued for 96 h. Hirudin: bolus of 0.1 mg/kg (maximum 15 mg), followed by a continuous infusion of 0.1 mg/kg/h (maximum 15 mg/h). Heparin: a bolus of 5000 U, followed by continuous infusion of 1000 U/h. Target aPTT 55 to 85 sec.

TIMI 9B

Thrombolysis and Thrombin Inhibition in Myocardial Infarction 9B

(continued)

Additional therapy

Intravenous thrombolytic therapy by the treating physician (front loaded tPA (maximum 100 mg) over 90 min or streptokinase, 1.5 million units over 1 h. Aspirin 150 to 325 mg/d. β blockers, nitrates, calcium channel blockers, and other medications were permitted.

Results

The hirudin-treated patients were more likely to have an aPTT within the target range ($p<0.0001$). Only 15% of the hirudin group vs 34% of the heparin group had aPTT values <55 sec within the first 24 h of therapy. The primary end-point of death, recurrent myocardial infarction, severe heart failure or cardiogenic shock by 30 days occurred in 11.9% of the heparin-treated group vs 12.9% of the hirudin-treated patients (p=NS). After adjustment for age, time to therapy, and type of thrombolytic therapy administered, there was no significant difference between the groups concerning occurrence of the primary end-point or in the occurrence of the individual elements of the composite end-point. Kaplan-Meier plots of the time to development of the composite endpoint and to the occurrence of death or reinfarction were comparable between the groups. Subgroup analyses could not identify a subgroup that clearly benefited from hirudin compared with heparin therapy. Major hemorrhage occurred in 5.3% of the heparin and 4.6% of the hirudin groups (p=NS), whereas intracranial hemorrhage in 0.9% vs 0.4%, respectively.

Conclusions

Hirudin had no treatment benefit over heparin in patients with acute myocardial infarction that received intravenous thrombolytic therapy.

IMPACT-AMI

Integrelin to Manage Platelet Aggregation to Combat Thrombosis

Title	Combined accelerated tissue-plasminogen activator and platelet glycoprotein IIb/IIIa integrin receptor blockade with integrilin in acute myocardial infarction. Results of a randomized, placebo-controlled, dose-ranging trial.
Authors	Ohman EM, Kleiman NS, Gacioch G, et al.
Reference	Circulation 1997;95:846-854.
Disease	Acute myocardial infarction.
Purpose	To evaluate the effects of platelet inhibition by integrilin on reperfusion, bleeding, and clinical outcome of patients with acute myocardial infarction treated with accelerated alteplase (tPA), heparin and aspirin.
Design	Placebo-controlled, dose-ranging, multicenter.
Patients	180 patients, 18 to 75 years old, within 6 hours of onset of acute myocardial infarction. Patients >125 kg, bleeding diathesis, severe hypertension, prior stroke, current warfarin therapy, anemia, thrombocytopenia, renal failure, recent noncompressible vascular puncture, ≥10 min cardiopulmonary resuscitation within 2 weeks, severe trauma within 6 months, or vasculitis were excluded.
Follow-up	Continuous 12-lead digital ECG for the first 24 h. Coronary angiography at 90 min after initiation of thrombolytic therapy. Clinical follow-up for in-hospital events.
Treatment regimen	Patients were enrolled in one of seven treatment groups of integrilin or placebo. Integrilin or placebo was administered within 10 min of initiation of alteplase.

IMPACT-AMI

Integrelin to Manage Platelet Aggregation to Combat Thrombosis

(continued)

Additional therapy

All patients received accelerated dose of alteplase IV (maximum dose 100 mg), and aspirin 325 mg/d. All but two groups received intravenous heparin. Target aPTT 2-2.5 times the control value.

Results

55 patients received placebo and 125 patients received integrilin. Of the 170 patients with adequate 90 min angiograms, patients allocated to the highest integrilin dose more often had complete reperfusion (TIMI flow grade III) than the placebo group (66% vs 39%, p=0.006). The rate of TIMI flow grade II or III was 87% vs 69%, respectively (p=0.01). The median time from initiation of thrombolytic therapy to steady-state recovery of ST segment deviation was 95 min for all integrilin-treated patients vs 116 min for the placebo-treated patients (p = 0.5). The duration was 65 min for the highest integrilin dose (p=0.05). 5.6% of the integrilin-treated patients vs 3.6% of the placebo-treated patients died (p=0.57). Death or reinfarction occured in 8.0% vs. 7.3%, respectively (p=0.87). The composite end-point of death, reinfarction, stroke, revascularization, or new in-hospital heart failure of pulmonary edema occurred in 45% of the integrilin (43% of the patients at the highest integrillin dose) vs 42% of the placebo-treated patients (p=0.71). Sustained hypotension occurred in 13% vs 16% respectively (p=0.53). Severe bleeding complications occurred in 2% of the integrilin-treated patients vs 5% of the placebo-treated patients, whereas moderate bleeding occurred in 14% vs 9% and mild bleeding in 63% vs 67% respectively.

Conclusions

Integrilin, when combined with alteplase, aspirin and heparin, accelerated the speed of reperfusion. However, integrilin therapy was not associated with improved in-hospital outcome.

1. Acute Myocardial Infarction

d. Early Versus Late Intervention After Acute Myocardial Infarction

TAMI

Thrombolysis and Angioplasty in Myocardial Infarction

Title	A randomized trial of immediate versus delayed elective angioplasty after intravenous tissue plasminogen activator in acute myocardial infarction.
Authors	Topol EJ, Califf RM, George BS, et al.
Reference	N Engl J Med 1987;317:581-588.
Disease	Acute myocardial infarction.
Purpose	To compare the efficacy of immediate versus delayed (7-10 days) coronary angioplasty in patients with acute myocardial infarction treated with intravenous tissue plasminogen activator.
Design	Randomized, open label, multicenter.
Patients	386 patients, age ≤75 years, with acute myocardial infarction < 4h from onset of symptoms (<6 h if severe ongoing pain was present) with ST≥1 mm in ≥2 leads. Only patients with TIMI grade 2-3 and ≥50% residual stenosis suitable to angioplasty 90 min after initiation of thrombolytic therapy, without ≥50% left main stenosis or left main equivalent stenosis were included (n=197).
Follow-up	7 days.
Treatment regimen	Immediate angioplasty or deferred elective angioplasty 5-10 days later.
Additional therapy	Tissue plasminogen activator (t-PA) 150 mg over 6-8 h (60-90 mg over the first h (10% of this as a bolus), heparin 5000 U IV and 500-1000 U/h ≥24 h, aspirin 325 mg/d, dipyridamole 75 mg X3/d, and diltiazem 30-60 mg X4/d.

TAMI

Thrombolysis and Angioplasty in Myocardial Infarction

(continued)

Results

Bleeding complications were common (18% of patients needed transfusion). The incidence of reocclusion was similar in the immediate (11%) and delayed (13%) angioplasty. Global and regional left ventricular function were comparable. The mortality was higher in the immediate (4.0%) than delayed (1.0%) angioplasty (p=0.37). 7% and 2% of the immediate and elective angioplasty groups needed emergency CABG (p=0.17), while 5% and 16% needed emergency angioplasty, respectively (p=0.01).

Conclusions

In patients with acute myocardial infarction and initially successful thrombolysis, immediate angioplasty offers no advantage over delayed elective angioplasty.

TIMI 2-A

Thrombolysis in Myocardial Infarction Trial (phase 2A)

Title

a. Immediate vs delayed catheterization and angioplasty following thrombolytic therapy for acute myocardial infarction. TIMI II-A results.
b. Comparison of immediate invasive, delayed invasive, and conservative strategies after tissue-type plasminogen activator. Results of the Thrombolysis in Myocardial Infarction (TIMI) phase II-A Trial.

Authors

a. The TIMI research group.
b. Rogers WJ, Baim DS, Gore JM, et al.

Reference

JAMA 1988;260:2849-2858.
Circulation 1990;81:1457-1476.

Disease

Acute myocardial infarction.

Purpose

To compare the results of three strategies of coronary angiography and angioplasty following intravenous thrombolytic therapy for acute myocardial infarction: immediate invasive, delayed invasive (18-48 h), and a conservative strategy.

Design

Randomized, open label, multicenter.

Patients

586 patients with acute myocardial infarction <76 years old < 4 hours from onset of symptoms with chest pain>30 min and ST elevation ≥0.1 mV in ≥2 contiguous leads.

Follow-up

Predischarge contrast ventriculography and coronary angiography. One-year follow-up.

TIMI 2-A

Thrombolysis in Myocardial Infarction Trial (phase 2A)

(continued)

Treatment regimen

1. Coronary angiography within 2 h of rt-PA initiation. PTCA was attempted if coronary anatomy was suitable.
2. Coronary angiography within 18-48 h of rt-PA initiation. PTCA was attempted if coronary anatomy was suitable.
3 Conservative strategy: coronary angiography and intervention only in those who had either spontaneous recurrent ischemia or a positive exercise test.

Additional therapy

Intravenous rt-PA (150 mg over 6 h for the first 520 patients, and 100 mg in the remaining 2742 patients). Lidocaine (1-1.5 mg/kg bolus + infusion 2-4 mg/min) for >24 h; heparin 5000 U bolus and infusion 1000 U/h for 5 days, and then subcutaneous until discharge. Aspirin 81 mg/d for 6 days and then 325 mg/d. Nifedipine 10-20 mg X3/d was administrated for 96 h. Metoprolol was started before discharge for one year.

Results

Predischarge contrast left ventricular ejection fraction was similar among the three groups. The rates of patency of the infarct related artery at the time of predischarge were similar among groups. However, the mean residual stenosis was greater in the conservative therapy arm (67.2%) than in the immediate invasive (50.6%) and delayed invasive (47.8%) arms ($p<0.001$). Immediate invasive strategy led to a higher rate of coronary artery bypass graft surgery after angioplasty (7.7%) than in the delayed invasive (2.1%) and conservative (2.5%) arms ($p<0.01$). The need for blood transfusion was greater in the immediate invasive (13.8%) than in the delayed invasive (3.1%) and conservative (2.0%) groups ($p<0.001$). One year mortality and reinfarction rates were similar among the three groups.

Conclusions

Conservative strategy achieves equally good results with less morbidity compared to invasive strategies.

TIMI 2

Thrombolysis in Myocardial Infarction Trial (phase 2)

Title	a. Comparison of invasive and conservative strategies after treatment with intravenous tissue plasminogen activator in acute myocardial infarction. Results of the Thrombolysis in Myocardial Infarction (TIMI) Phase II Trial. b. One-year results of the Thrombolysis in Myocardial Infarction investigation (TIMI) phase II trial.
Authors	a. The TIMI Study Group. b. Williams DO, Braunwald E, Knatterud G, et al.
Reference	a. N Engl J Med 1989;320:618-627. b. Circulation 1992;85:533-542.
Disease	Acute myocardial infarction.
Purpose	To compare an invasive strategy consisting of coronary angiography and angioplasty within 18-48 h of infarction and a conservative approach in which angiography was performed only in patients with spontaneous or exercise induced ischemia in patients with acute myocardial infarction treated with rt-PA.
Design	Randomized, open label, multicenter.
Patients	3262 patients with acute myocardial infarction <76 years old < 4 hours from onset of symptoms with chest pain>30 min and ST elevation ≥0.1 mV in ≥2 contiguous leads.
Follow-up	a. Predischarge radionuclide ventriculography at rest and during exercise. At six weeks clinical evaluation and maximal exercise test + radionuclide ventriculography. b. One year.

TIMI 2

Thrombolysis in Myocardial Infarction Trial (phase 2)

(continued)

Treatment regimen Coronary angiography and angioplasty (if arteriography demonstrated suitable anatomy) within 18-48 h of thrombolytic therapy versus coronary angiography only for patients who had either spontaneous recurrent ischemia or a positive exercise test (the conservative arm).

Additional therapy Intravenous rt-PA (150 mg over 6 h for the first 520 patients, and 100 mg in the remaining 2742 patients). Lidocaine (1-1.5 mg/kg bolus + infusion 2-4 mg/min) for >24 h; heparin 5000 U bolus and infusion 1000 U/h for 5 days, and then subcutaneous until discharge. Aspirin 80 mg/d for 6 days and then 325 mg/d

---

Results a. 53.7% and 13.3% of the invasive strategy and conservative groups underwent angioplasty within 14 days of admission. Reinfarction or death within 6 weeks occurred in 10.9% and 9.7% of the invasive and conservative group, respectively (p=0.25). Predischarge and 6-week left ventricular ejection fraction at either rest or during exercise were comparable.
b. Death or nonfatal reinfarction within 1 year occurred in 14.7% and 15.2% of the invasive and conservative groups, respectively. There was no difference in death or recurrent infarction rates between the 2 groups. Anginal status at 1 year was comparable. Cardiac catheterization and angioplasty were performed more often in the invasive group (98% and 61.2%) versus the conservative group (45.2% and 20.5%). In patients with prior infarction, six weeks and one year mortality was lower in the invasive group (6.0% and 10.3%) than in the conservative group (11.5% and 17.0%), p= 0.04 and p=0.03, respectively.

Conclusions In patients with acute myocardial infarction who are treated with rt-PA, heparin and aspirin, the results of an invasive and conservative strategies are comparable.

SWIFT

Should We Intervene Following Thrombolysis?

Title	SWIFT trial of delayed elective intervention vs conservative treatment after thrombolysis with anistreplase in acute myocardial infarction.
Authors	SWIFT Trial Study Group.
Reference	Br Med J 1991;302:555-560.
Disease	Acute myocardial infarction.
Purpose	To compare a strategy of conservative management to early elective angiography and intervention following thrombolytic therapy for acute myocardial infarction.
Design	Randomized, open label, multicenter.
Patients	800 patients, <70 years of age, with clinical features of first acute myocardial infarction, ≤3 h from onset of symptoms, and ST elevation >1 mm in ≥2 limb leads or >2 mm in ≥2 precordial leads. Patients with cardiogenic shock, severe hypertension, or contraindication to thrombolytic therapy were excluded.
Follow-up	12 month clinical follow-up. Radionuclide left ventriculography 2-3 months (523 patients) and 12 months (492 patients) after randomization.
Treatment regimen	1. Coronary angiography within 48 h. Angioplasty was attempted for >50% residual stenosis. 2. Conservative management. Angiography was permitted for persisting or recurrent ischemia or after a positive exercise test.

SWIFT

Should We Intervene Following Thrombolysis?

Additional therapy Anistreplase 30 U IV over 5 min. Heparin infusion 1000 U/h was started 4-6 h later. Oral anticoagulation was optional. Oral ß blocker (timolol).

Results 43% of the early angiography group underwent angioplasty and 15% had coronary artery bypass grafting during the initial hospitalization. 3% of the conservative group had angioplasty and 2% bypass surgery. The median length of hospitalization was 11 and 10 days in the intervention and conservative groups (p<0.0001). 27% of the intervention group and 14% of the conservative group were in the hospital for >14 day. More patients in the conservative group underwent interventions during the 1 year follow-up. In-hospital mortality was 2.7% vs 3.3% in the conservative and intervention groups. One year mortality was 5.0% vs 5.8%, respectively (OR 1.18, 95% CI 0.64-2.10, p=0.64). In-hospital reinfarction occurred in 8.2% vs 12.1%, respectively, while reinfarction by 11 months was 15.1% vs 12.9% (OR 1.16, 95% CI 0.77-1.75, p=0.42). Angina at rest after 12 months occurred in 6.3% vs 3.4%, respectively (p=NS). The left ventricular ejection fraction at 2-3 and 12 months were comparable between the two groups.

Conclusions There is no advantage for early routine intervention over a conservative approach following intravenous thrombolytic therapy for acute myocardial infarction.

1. Acute Myocardial Infarction
e. Remodeling After Infarction

SAVE

Survival and Ventricular Enlargement

Title	a. Rationale, design and baseline characteristics of the survival and ventricular enlargement trial. b. Effect of captopril on mortality and morbidity in patients with left ventricular dysfunction after myocardial infarction. Results of the Survival and Ventricular Enlargement trial.
Authors	a. Moyé LA, Pfeffer MA, Braunwald E, et al. b. Pfeffer MA, Braunwald E, Moyé LA, et al.
Reference	a. Am J Cardiol 1991;68:70D-79D. b. N Engl J Med 1992;327:669-677.
Disease	Acute myocardial infarction.
Purpose	To investigate whether captopril could reduce mortality and morbidity in patients with left ventricular dysfunction following myocardial infarction.
Design	Randomized, double blind, placebo controlled, multicenter.
Patients	2231 patients, 21-80 years of age, 3-16 days after myocardial infarction with left ventricular ejection fraction ≤40%, but without active ischemia or overt heart failure.
Follow-up	Clinical follow-up for 24-60 months (average 42 months). Radionuclide ventriculogram at baseline and an average of 36 months later.
Treatment regimen	Captopril (initial dose 12.5 mg. Dose was increased gradually to 50 mg X3/d), or placebo.

SAVE

Survival and Ventricular Enlargement

(continued)

Results

Total mortality was lower in the captopril group (20% vs 25%, risk reduction 19%, 95% CI 3-32%, p=0.019). The reduction of risk for cardiovascular mortality was 21% (95% CI 5-35%, p=0.014). The reduction in the risk of death from progressive heart failure was 36% (95% CI 4-58%, p=0.032). Progressive heart failure unresponsive to digitalis and diuretics developed in 11% of the captopril and 16% of the placebo patients (risk reduction 37%, 95% CI 20-50%, p<0.001). Recurrent myocardial infraction was experienced by 15.2% of the placebo and 11.9% of the captopril group (risk reduction 25%, 95% CI 5-40%, p=0.015). Deterioration of ≥9 units in left ventricular ejection fraction was detected in 16% of the placebo and 13% of the captopril group (p=0.17).

Conclusions

Long term captopril therapy in patients with asymptomatic left ventricular dysfunction following acute myocardial infarction was associated with lower mortality and morbidity. These benefits were observed in patients who received thrombolytic therapy aspirin, or ß blockers, as well as those who did not.

CONSENSUS II

Cooperative New Scandinavian Enalapril Survival Study II

Title	Effects of the early administration of enalapril on mortality in patients with acute myocardial infarction. Results of the Cooperative New Scandinavian Enalapril Survival Study II (CONSENSUS II).
Authors	Swedberg K, Held P, Kjekhus J, et al.
Reference	N Engl J Med 1992;327:678-684.
Disease	Acute myocardial infarction.
Purpose	To evaluate whether early administration of enalapril after acute myocardial infarction would reduce mortality during the 6 months follow-up.
Design	Randomized, double blind, placebo controlled, multicenter.
Patients	6090 patients within 24 h of onset of pain, with ST elevation in ≥2 leads, or new Q waves, or elevated levels of enzymes. Patients with supine blood pressure less than 105/65 mmHg were excluded.
Follow-up	41-180 days of follow-up.
Treatment regimen	IV infusion of 1mg enalaprilat or placebo over 2h. If blood pressure declined <90/60 mmHg, the infusion was stopped temporarily. 6 h later, oral enalapril or placebo was started. The recommended starting dose was 2.5 mg X2/d with gradual increase up to 20 mg/d.
Additional therapy	Standard therapy including nitrates, ß blockers, calcium channel blockers, thrombolytic therapy, aspirin, anticoagulants, and diuretics, as indicated. If a patient needed angiotensin converting enzyme for heart failure, the patient was withdrawn from the study.

Results

The trial was terminated prematurely by the safety committee. By the end of the trial the mortality was 9.4% vs 10.2% in the placebo and enalapril groups (p=0.26). The mortality rates according to life-table analysis at 10 days and at 1, 3, and 6 months were 4.3% vs 4.6%, 6.3% vs 7.2%, 8.2% vs 9.1%, and 10.2% vs 11.0%, respectively (p=0.26). The relative risk associated with enalapril therapy was 1.10 (95% CI 0.93-1.29). Death due to progressive heart failure occurred in 3.4% and 4.3% of the placebo and enalapril groups, whereas there was no difference in sudden death, death due to myocardial rupture, or stroke. 30% of the placebo and 27% of the enalapril treated patients needed change of therapy due to heart failure (p<0.006). Reinfarction occurred in 9% of the patients in each group. Early hypotension (systolic blood pressure <90 mmHg, or diastolic blood pressure <50 mmHg) occurred in 3% of the control and 12% of the enalapril patients (p<0.001).

Conclusions

Enalapril therapy, started within 24 h of the onset of acute myocardial infarction did not improve survival during the 180 days of follow-up.

AIRE

The Acute Infarction Ramipril Efficacy

Title	a. The acute infarction ramipril efficacy (AIRE) study: rationale, design, organization, and outcome definitions. b. Effect of ramipril on mortality and morbidity of survivors of acute myocardial infarction with clinical evidence of heart failure.
Authors	a. Hall AS, Winter C, Bogie SM, et al. b. The AIRE Study Investigators.
Reference	a. J Cardiovasc Pharmacol 1991;18(Suppl 2):S105-S109. b. Lancet 1993;342:821-828.
Disease	Acute myocardial infarction. Heart failure.
Purpose	To determine whether early oral treatment with ramipril will reduce mortality in patients with heart failure complicating acute myocardial infarction.
Design	Randomized, double blind, placebo controlled. multicenter.
Patients	1986 patients, aged ≥18 years, with a definite myocardial infarction and signs of heart failure (even transient) in some period after the infarction. Patients with heart failure due to valvular heart disease, unstable angina, severe and resistant heart failure, or contraindications to angiotensin converting enzyme inhibition were excluded.
Follow-up	Clinical follow-up for >6 months (average 15 months).
Treatment regimen	3-10 days following infarction patients were randomized to receive ramipril 2.5 mg or placebo. The dose was increased to 5 mg X2/d (or 2.5 mg X2/d in case of intolerance).
Additional therapy	Patients could continue or begin any other medication except an angiotensin converting enzyme inhibitor.

AIRE

The Acute Infarction Ramipril Efficacy

(continued)

Results

Total mortality was 17% in the ramipril and 23% in the placebo group (27% risk reduction, 95% CI 11%-40%, p=0.002). Separation of the survival curves occurred very early (within 30 days) and continued to diverge throughout the study. Severe heart failure developed in 14% vs 18% respectively. There was no difference in the rates of stroke and reinfarction between the groups. Death, severe heart failure, myocardial infarction, or stroke developed in 28% vs 34% of the ramipril and placebo group (risk reduction 19%, 95% CI 5%-31%, p=0.008). Reported serious adverse events occurred in 58% of the ramipril vs 64% of the placebo. There was no difference in the occurrence of renal failure, angina or syncope.

Conclusions

Ramipril therapy, started 3-10 days after infarction in patients with persistent or transient heart failure following infarction resulted in reduction of mortality.

GISSI-3

Gruppo Italiano per lo Studio della Sopravvivenza nell'Infarto Miocardico III

Title	a. GISSI-3: effect of lisinopril and transdermal glyceryl trinitrate singly and together on 6-week mortality and ventricular function after acute myocardial infarction. b. Six-month effects of early treatment with lisinopril and transdermal glyceryl trinitrate singly and together withdrawn six weeks after acute myocardial infarction: the GISSI-3 trial.
Authors	GISSI.
Reference	a. Lancet 1994;343:1115-1122. b. J Am Coll Cardiol 1996;27:337-344.
Disease	Acute myocardial infarction.
Purpose	To evaluate the efficacy of lisinopril, transdermal glyceryl trinitrate, and their combination on survival and left ventricular function following acute myocardial infarction.
Design	Randomized, open label, 2X2 factorial, multicenter.
Patients	18895 patients with chest pain, 24 h of onset of symptoms, and ST elevation or depression of ≥1 mm in ≥1 limb lead, or ≥2 mm in ≥1 precordial lead. Patients with severe heart failure, or contraindication to medications were excluded.
Follow-up	6 month clinical follow-up. Echocardiography at 6 weeks (14,209 patients).
Treatment regimen	1. Oral lisinopril 5 mg at randomization and 10 mg/d for 6 weeks, or open control. 2. Glyceryl trinitrate (GTN) IV for 24 h, started at a rate of 5 μg/min and increased until systolic blood pressure fell by 10% or below 90 mmHg. >24 h transdermal GTN 10 mg/d for 14 h each day for 6 weeks, or placebo.

Additional therapy Recommended therapy included thrombolysis (72% of the patients), oral aspirin (84%), and IV β blockers (31%).

Results 13.3% of the control patients received non-study ACE inhibitors. The 6 week mortality was 6.3% and 7.1% in the lisinopril and control groups (OR 0.88, 95% CI 0.79-0.99, p=0.03). The survival curve separated on the first day and continued to diverge throughout the 6-weeks. The combined end point of mortality, heart failure beyond day 4 of infarction, left ventricular ejection fraction ≤35%, or ≥45% myocardial segments with abnormal motion occurred in 15.6% and 17.0% (OR 0.90, 95% CI 0.84-0.98, p=0.009). Rates of recurrent infarction, post-infarction angina, cardiogenic shock, and stroke were similar between the lisinopril and control groups. 57.1% of the patients that were not assigned to GTN received nitrates (11.3% for >5 days). GTN did not alter total mortality (6.5% vs 6.9%, p=0.28), or the combined end point (15.9% vs 16.7%, p=0.12). The GTN group had lower rate of post-infarction angina (20.0% vs 21.2%, OR 0.93, 95% CI 0.86-0.99, p=0.033), and cardiogenic shock (2.1.% vs 2.6%, OR 0.78, 95% CI 0.64-0.94, p=0.009). However, the rate of stroke was higher with GTN (0.9% vs 0.6%, p=0.027). After 6 months 18.1% vs 19.3% of the lisinopril and control groups developed severe left ventricular dysfunction or died (p=0.03), while 5.4% vs 5.8% developed clinical heart failure. No differences were found between patients with and without GTN, after 6 months.

Conclusions 6 week lisinopril therapy reduced mortality and improved outcome after myocardial infarction. There is no evidence that GTN altered these outcomes significantly.

ISIS-4

International Study of Infarct Survival

Title	ISIS-4: a randomized factorial trial assessing early oral captopril, oral mononitrate, and intravenous magnesium sulphate in 58050 patients with suspected acute myocardial infarction.
Authors	ISIS-4 (Fourth International Study of Infarct Survival) Collaborative Group.
Reference	Lancet 1995;345:669-685.
Disease	Acute myocardial infarction.
Purpose	To assess the effects on major morbidity and 5-week mortality in patients with suspected acute myocardial infarction of early initiation of oral captopril, oral controlled-release mononitrate, and intravenous magnesium sulphate.
Design	Randomized double-blind, placebo controlled (captopril and mononitrate); randomized (magnesium versus open control), multicenter.
Patients	58,050 patients with suspected infarction admitted within 24 hours of onset of symptoms with no clear indications for, or contraindications to, the study medications. Patients that received nitrates for only a few days were included.
Follow-up	Clinical follow-up for 5 weeks (97% of the patients); one year (68% of the patients).

ISIS-4

International Study of Infarct Survival

(continued)

Treatment regimen

1. Patients were randomized to oral captopril or placebo (6.25 mg initially; 12.5 mg 2 hours later; 25 mg 10-12 hours later; and thereafter 50 mg BID for 28 days).
2. Patients received either oral mononitrate or placebo (30 mg upon randomization and after 10-12 hours; 60 mg/d for 28 days).
3. Half the patients receive intravenous magnesium sulfate (8 mmol as a bolus over 15 min and then 72 mmol over 24 hours).

Additional therapy

Antiplatelet therapy was recommended (received by 94% of patients). 70% of the patients received thrombolytic therapy.

Results

Analysis was by intention to treat. Captopril reduced 5-week mortality by 7% (95% CI of 13% to 1% reduction; p=0.02) (7.19% versus 7.69%, in the captopril and placebo groups, respectively). Mononitrate therapy did not alter 5-week mortality (7.34% versus 7.54% in the treated and control groups, respectively). Intravenous magnesium therapy did not reduce 5-week mortality (7.64% versus 7.24% in the magnesium and control groups, respectively).

Conclusions

Oral captopril , started early upon admission reduces 5-week mortality in patients with suspected acute myocardial infarction. Oral mononitrate or intravenous magnesium sulfate did not reduce mortality.

SMILE

Survival of Myocardial Infarction Long-Term Evaluation

Title	The effect of the angiotensin-converting-enzyme inhibitor zofenopril on mortality and morbidity after anterior myocardial infarction..
Authors	Ambrosioni E, Borghi C, Magnani B, for the Survival of Myocardial Infarction Long-Term Evaluation (SMILE) Study Investigators.
Reference	N Engl L Med 1995;332:80-85.
Disease	Anterior wall acute myocardial infarction.
Purpose	To evaluate whether 6 weeks of therapy with angiotensin-converting-enzyme inhibitor zofenopril, started within 24 hours after onset of infarction will improve short and long term outcome.
Design	Randomized, placebo controlled, multicenter.
Patients	1556 patients with anterior wall acute myocardial infarction who did not receive reperfusion therapy. (772 and 784 patients received zofenopril and placebo, respectively).
Follow-up	Clinical follow-up for 1-year.
Treatment regimen	Oral zofenopril 7.5 mg initially, and 12 hours later. The dose was increased gradually to 30 mg BID if SBP>100 mmHg and there were no signs or symptoms of hypotension. Patients unable to tolerate the first dose were withdrawn from the study but included in the intention to treat analysis. Treatment was continued for six weeks.

Results

Six weeks after randomization, the zofenopril treated patients had a 46% reduction in the risk of severe congestive heart failure (95% CI 11-71%; p=0.018) and 25% reduction in mortality rate (95% CI -11-60%; p=0.19). The incidence of severe heart failure and death were 4.1% and 6.5% for the placebo group and 2.2% and 4.9% for the zofenopril group, respectively. The one-year mortality was lower in the zofenopril treated group (10.0%) than in the control (14.1%) (29% risk reduction; 95% CI 6-51%; p=0.011)

Conclusions

Six weeks of therapy with zofenopril, started within 24 hours after onset of myocardial infarction, reduced six week and one-year mortality and reduced the incidence of severe heart failure in patients with anterior wall acute myocardial infarction not receiving reperfusion therapy.

TRACE

Trandolapril Cardiac Evaluation

Title	A clinical trial of the angiotensin-converting-enzyme inhibitor trandolapril in patients with left ventricular dysfunction after myocardial infarction.
Authors	Køber L, Torp-Pedersen C, Clarsen JE, et al.
Reference	N Engl J Med 1995;333:1670-1676.
Disease	Congestive heart failure, myocardial infarction.
Purpose	To determine whether patients with left ventricular dysfunction soon after myocardial infarction benefit from long-term oral ACE inhibition.
Design	Randomized, double blind, placebo controlled, multicenter.
Patients	1749 patients, >18 years old, who survived acute myocardial infarction 2-6 days earlier. Only patients with echocardiographic proof of left ventricular dysfunction (wall-motion index ≤1.2) without contraindication or definite need for ACE inhibition were included.
Follow-up	24-50 months.
Treatment regimen	3-7 days after infarction patients were randomized to trandolapril 1 mg/d or placebo. The dose was gradually increased to 1-4 mg/d.
Additional therapy	Aspirin, ß blockers, calcium antagonists, diuretics, nitrates, and digoxin, as clinically indicated.

TRACE

Trandolapril Cardiac Evaluation

(continued)

Results

Total mortality after 4 year was 34.7% in the trandolapril group and 42.3% in the placebo group. The relative risk of death from any cause for the treated versus placebo groups was 0.78 (95% CI 0.67-0.91, p=0.001). The mortality curves diverged early and continued to diverge throughout the follow-up period. Cardiovascular death occurred in 25.8% and 33.0% of the trandolapril and placebo groups (RR 0.75, 95% CI 0.63-0.89, p=0.001). Trandolapril also reduced the rate of sudden death (RR 0.76, 95% CI 0.59-0.98, p=0.03), and the progression to severe heart failure (RR 0.71, 95% CI 0.56-0.89, p=0.003). There was a trend towards reduction of recurrent infarction with trandolapril (RR 0.86, 95% CI 0.66-1.13, p=0.29).

Conclusions

Long term treatment with trandolapril in patients with left ventricular dysfunction soon after myocardial infarction reduces the rates of death, cardiovascular mortality, sudden death, and progression to severe heart failure.

CATS

Captopril And Thrombolysis Study

Title a. Acute intervention with captopril during thrombolysis in patients with first anterior myocardial infarction. Results from the captopril and thrombolysis study (CATS). b. Which patient benefits from early angiotensin-converting enzyme inhibition after myocardial infarction? Results of one-year serial echocardiographic follow-up from the captopril and thrombolysis study (CATS).

Authors a. Kingma JH, van Gilst WH, Peels KH, et al.
b. Van Gilst WH, Kingma H, Peels KH, et al.

Reference a. Eur Heart J 1994;15:898-907.
b. J Am Coll Cardiol 1996;28:114-121

Disease Acute myocardial infarction.

Purpose To evaluate the effects of early captopril therapy (within 6 h of onset of first anterior myocardial infarction) on left ventricular volume and clinical symptoms.

Design Multicenter, randomized, double blind, placebo-controlled.

Patients 298 patients with first anterior acute myocardial infarction treated with streptokinase <6h of onset of symptoms. Patients with systolic blood pressure >200 or <100 mmHg or diastolic blood pressure >120 or <55 mmHg were excluded. Patients with renal insufficiency or intolerance to angiotensin converting enzyme inhibitors, severe valvular heart disease, arrhythmias requiring antiarrhythmic therapy, serious systemic disease, AV conduction disturbances, or left bundle branch block were excluded.

Follow-up 12 months clinical 24h ambulatory ECG monitoring, and echocardiographic follow-up.

CATS

Captopril And Thrombolysis Study

(continued)

Treatment regimen

Immediately upon completion of streptokinase, captopril (6.25 mg) or placebo was given PO. The dose was repeated after 4 and 8h. Captopril 12.5 mg and 25 mg were given at 16h and 24h, respectively. If systolic blood pressure was <95 mmHg, the study medication was withheld until the next dosing time. The target dose was 25 mgX3/d.

Additional therapy

IV Streptokinase 1.5 million IU over 30 min. Aspirin, calcium antagonists and β-blockers were at the discretion of the local investigators.

Results

In the captopril group the number of patients with paired ventricular premature beats, accelerated idioventricular rhythm and non-sustained ventricular tachycardia were lower than in the placebo group. During the acute phase accelerated idioventricular rhythm occurred in 33.8% vs 44.5%, in the captopril and placebo group ($p<0.05$), and non-sustained ventricular tachycardia in 31.7% vs 40.9%, respectively ($p<0.05$). Peak creatine kinase and cumulative α-hydroxybutyrate dehydrogenase release over 72h tended to be lower, and peak α-hydroxybutyrate dehydrogenase was lower in the captopril group than in the placebo group. A complete clinical follow-up over 1 year was obtained in 245 patients (82.2%). Analysis with the random coefficient model revealed no significant effect of captopril on changes in left ventricular volume over 12 months when compared with placebo. However, the occurrence of dilatation was lower in the captopril-treated group ($p=0.018$). Captopril was effective in reducing the occurrence of dilatation in medium size infarcts, tended to be effective in small infarcts, but was ineffective in large infarcts. The incidence of heart failure was lower in the captopril group ($p<0.04$). This effect was confined to patients with medium size infarctions.

Conclusions

Very early treatment with captopril reduces the occurrence of early dilatation and progression to heart failure, especially in patients with medium-size infarction.

1. Acute Myocardial Infarction
f. Miscellaneous

TIMI 2-B

Thrombolysis in Myocardial Infarction Trial (phase 2B)

Title a. Comparison of invasive and conservative strategies after treatment with intravenous tissue plasminogen activator in acute myocardial infarction. Results of the Thrombolysis in Myocardial Infarction (TIMI) Phase II Trial.
b. Immediate versus deferred ß-blockade following thrombolytic therapy in patients with acute myocardial infarction. Results of the Thrombolysis in Myocardial Infarction (TIMI) II-B Study.

Authors a. The TIMI Study Group.
b. Roberts R, Rogers WJ, Mueller HS, et al.

Reference a. N Engl J Med 1989;320:618-627.
b. Circulation 1991;83:422-437.

Disease Acute myocardial infarction.

Purpose To compare the effects of immediate versus delayed (6 days) metoprolol therapy in patients with acute myocardial infarction treated with rt-PA (a substudy of the TIMI-2 Trial).

Design Randomized, open label, multicenter study.

Patients 2948 patients with acute myocardial infarction <76 years old < 4 hours from onset of symptoms with chest pain>30 min and ST elevation ≥0.1 mV in ≥2 contiguous leads, of whom 1434 (49%) were eligible for ß-blocker therapy.

Follow-up Predischarge radionuclide ventriculography at rest and during exercise. At six weeks clinical evaluation and maximal exercise test + radionuclide ventriculography. One-year follow-up.

Treatment regimen Immediate therapy: 3 IV injections of 5 mg metoprolol, and then 50 mg X2/d PO for 1 day and 100 mg X2/d thereafter. Delayed therapy: on day 6, 50 mg X2/d PO for one day and then 100 mg X2/d.

Thrombolysis in Myocardial Infarction Trial (phase 2B)

(continued)

Additional therapy Intravenous rt-PA (150 mg over 6 h for the first 520 patients, and 100 mg in the remaining 2742 patients). Lidocaine (1-1.5 mg/kg bolus + infusion 2-4 mg/min) for >24 h; heparin 5000 U bolus and infusion 1000 U/h for 5 days, and then subcutaneous until discharge. Aspirin 80 mg/d for 6 days and then 325 mg/d.

Results The systolic blood pressure in the immediate group decreased during the first hour by 9.8% compared with 7.1% in the deferred therapy group (P<0.01). Mean heart rate decreased by 6% in the immediate group and increased in the deferred group (P<0.001). There was no difference in the occurrence of arrhythmias between the groups. Left ventricular ejection fraction was similar in both groups at predischarge (51.0% versus 50.1%) and at 6 weeks (50.4% and 50.8%, respectively). Regional ventricular function was also comparable. Overall, there was no difference in mortality between the groups. However, in the low risk patients 6-weeks mortality was 0 and 2.8% in the immediate and deferred ß-blocker therapy groups (p=0.007). Reinfarction was less common at 6 days and 6 weeks in the immediate treated group. However, there was no difference at one year.

Conclusions ß-blockers are safe when given early after thrombolytic therapy to a selected population with acute myocardial infarction and are associated with lower risk of recurrent ischemia and reinfarction in the first week. However, long term prognosis and left ventricular function are similar to those who receive ß-blockers only after 6 days.

DAVIT II

The Danish Verapamil Infarction Trial II

Title	Effect of verapamil on mortality and major events after acute myocardial infarction (the Danish Verapamil Infarction Trial II- DAVIT II).
Authors	The Danish Study Group on Verapamil in Myocardial Infarction.
Reference	Am J Cardiol 1990;66:779-785.
Disease	Acute myocardial infarction.
Purpose	To assess whether long term therapy with verapamil, started from the second week after acute myocardial infarction will reduce mortality and morbidity compared with placebo.
Design	Randomized. double blind, placebo controlled, multicenter.
Patients	1775 patients, <76 years old, 7-15 days after proven acute myocardial infarction. Patients with severe heart failure, hypotension, atrioventricular or sinoatrial blocks, or therapy with calcium channel or ß blockers due to angina, arrhythmia, or hypertension were excluded.
Follow-up	Clinical follow-up up to 18 months (mean 16 months).
Treatment regimen	Verapamil 120 mg X3/d (in cases of adverse drug reactions 120 mg X1-2/d was allowed) or placebo.
Additional therapy	Therapy with calcium channel blockers or ß blockers was not permitted. Nitrates were allowed.

DAVIT II

The Danish Verapamil Infarction Trial II

(continued)

Results

1 month after randomization 38.7% of the placebo and 33.2% of the verapamil group reported angina (p=0.02). However, after 12 months, the difference did not reach statistical significance (33.7% vs 28.6%). There was a trend towards reduction of total mortality (11.1% vs 13.8%, Hazard ratio (HR) 0.80, 95% CI 0.61-1.05, p=0.11), and a significant reduction of death or first reinfarction (18.0% vs 21.6%, HR 0.80, 95% CI 0.64-0.99, p=0.03) at 18 months with verapamil. In patients without heart failure during hospitalization, verapamil was associated with lower mortality (7.7% vs 11.8%, HR 0.64, 95% CI 0.44-0.94, p=0.02) and reinfarction (9.4% vs 12.7%, HR 0.67, 95% CI 0.46-0.97, p=0.02), while there was no difference in mortality (17.5% vs 17.9%) or reinfarction (14.3% vs 14.2%) between the groups in patients with heart failure during hospitalization.

Conclusions

Long-term verapamil therapy after an acute myocardial infarction resulted in reduction of mortality and reinfarction, but only in patients without heart failure.

LIMIT-2

Leicester Intravenous Magnesium Intervention II Trial

Title	Intravenous magnesium sulphate in suspected acute myocardial infarction: results of the second Leicester Intravenous Magnesium Intervention Trial (LIMIT-2).
Authors	Woods KL, Fletcher S, Roffe C, Haider Y.
Reference	Lancet 1992;339:1553-1558.
Disease	Acute myocardial infarction.
Purpose	To evaluate the efficacy of intravenous magnesium sulphate infusion in reduction of early mortality following acute myocardial infarction.
Design	Randomized, double blind, placebo controlled, unicenter.
Patients	2316 patients with suspected acute myocardial infarction (within 24 h of onset of symptoms). No electrocardiographic criteria were specified.
Follow-up	28 days clinical follow-up.
Treatment regimen	Saline or magnesium sulphate 8 mmol over 5 min followed by 65 mmol over 24 h.
Additional therapy	No restriction. Thrombolytic therapy was not required.

LIMIT-2

Leicester Intravenous Magnesium Intervention II Trial

(continued)

Results

Acute myocardial infarction was confirmed in 65% of the patients. 36% vs 35% of the magnesium and placebo patients received thrombolytic therapy, while 65% vs 66% received aspirin. 28 day mortality was 10.3% in the placebo and 7.8% in the magnesium group (odds ratio 0.74, 95% CI 0.55-1.00, p=0.04). Mortality odds ratios were 0.76 (95% CI 0.46-1.27) in the patients that received thrombolytic therapy and 0.72 (95% CI 0.49-0.99) for those who did not receive thrombolytic therapy. The incidence of clinical left ventricular failure was 11.2% in the magnesium and 14.9% in the placebo group (25% risk reduction, 95% CI 7%-39%, p=0.009). The prevalence of hypotension <100 mmHg for ≥1 h was similar. Sinus bradycardia was more common with magnesium (10.8% vs 8.0%, p=0.02). However, the incidence of AV block and tachyarrhythmias were similar.

Conclusions

Intravenous magnesium sulphate is a simple and safe therapy for acute myocardial infarction and was associated with reduction of mortality.

ESPRIM

European Study of Prevention of Infarct with Molsidomine.

Title	The ESPRIM trial: short-term treatment of acute myocardial infarction with molsidomine.
Authors	European Study of Prevention of Infarct with Molsidomine (ESPRIM) Group.
Reference	Lancet 1994;344:91-97.
Disease	Acute myocardial infarction.
Purpose	To compare the effects of molsidomine (a nitric oxide donor) with placebo in patients with acute myocardial infarction.
Design	Randomized, double blind, placebo controlled, multicenter.
Patients	4017 patients with suspected acute myocardial infarction (chest pain >30 min, with onset <24 h). Patients in Killip class III or IV were excluded.
Follow-up	An average of 13 months clinical follow-up.
Treatment regimen	Molsidomine (IV linsidomine (the active metabolite of molsidomine) 1 mg/h for 48 h, followed by oral molsidomine 4 mg X4/d for 12 days. The control group received matching placebo
Additional therapy	Non-study vasodilator therapy could be added by the physician. No limitation on additional therapy

Results

48.5% of the molsidomine and 51.0% of the placebo received thrombolytic therapy before randomization, and 21.7% vs 20.0% after randomization. 35 day mortality was similar (8.4% vs 8.8% in the molsidomine and placebo groups, RR 0.96, 95% CI 0.78-1.17, p=0.66). There was no difference in long-term mortality 14.7% vs 14.2% in the molsidomine and placebo groups, respectively (p=0.67). The rates of the major and minor adverse events were similar, except for headache which was more common with the molsidomine group.

Conclusions

Nitric oxide donor was not effective in reduction of mortality following acute myocardial infarction.

TAMI-9

Thrombolysis and Angioplasty in Myocardial Infarction 9 Trial

Title	Intravenous fluosol in the treatment of acute myocardial infarction. Results of the thrombolysis and angioplasty in myocardial infarction 9 trial.
Authors	Wall TC, Califf RM, Blankenship J, et al.
Reference	Circulation 1994;90:114-120.
Disease	Acute myocardial infarction.
Purpose	To assess the efficacy of fluosol as an adjunctive therapy to reperfusion for acute myocardial infarction.
Design	Randomized, open label, multicenter.
Patients	430 patients, age >18 and <75 years, with suspected acute myocardial infarction <6h of onset of symptoms, with ≥1 mm ST elevation in ≥2 leads.
Follow-up	Cardiac angiography and symptom-limited stress thallium scan 5-14 days after infarction. In-hospital clinical follow-up.
Treatment regimen	IV fluosol 1 ml/min, the rate was increased gradually to 20 ml/min. Total dose 15 ml/kg.
Additional therapy	Chewable aspirin 324 mg, IV heparin, and 100 mg tissue plasminogen activator over 3 h, 100% oxygen for 8 h. IV atenolol if no contraindications existed.

Results

There was no significant difference between the control and fluosol groups in left ventricular ejection fraction (52% vs 51%), regional wall motion analysis (-2.2 SD/chord vs -2.4 SD/chord), or infarct size as measured by thallium scan. The analysis of anterior wall infarction yielded similar results. Patency rates of the infarct related arteries were similar. Rates of death (3.7% vs 5.6%) and stroke (0.9% vs 4.3%) were similar in the control and fluosol groups. However, the fluosol group experienced less recurrent infarction (4.2% vs 2.4%), but more heart failure and pulmonary edema (31% vs 45%; p=0.004). There was no difference in hemorrhagic complications.

Conclusions

Fluosol, as an adjunctive therapy to thrombolysis did not result in reduction of infarct size, or improvement of left ventricular function and clinical outcome.

DIGAMI

Diabetes Mellitus Insulin-Glucose Infusion in Acute Myocardial Infarction

Title	Randomized trial of insulin-glucose infusion followed by subcutaneous insulin treatment in diabetic patients with acute myocardial infarction (DIGAMI study): effects on mortality at 1 year.
Authors	Malmberg K, Rydén L, Efendic S, et al.
Reference	J Am Coll Cardiol 1995;26:57-65.
Disease	Acute myocardial infarction, diabetes mellitus.
Purpose	To evaluate whether insulin-glucose infusion followed by multidose insulin therapy will decrease mortality in diabetic patients with acute myocardial infarction.
Design	Randomized, open label, multicenter.
Patients	620 patients with diabetes mellitus and a blood glucose level>11 mmol/l and with suspected acute myocardial infarction (chest pain of ≥15 min, ≤24 h of onset of symptoms).
Follow-up	1 year.
Treatment regimen	Insulin-glucose or placebo infusion over ≥24 h, then SC insulin X4/d for ≥3 months.
Additional therapy	Thrombolytic therapy, if no contraindications existed and patients were admitted within 6 h of onset of symptoms. IV followed by oral metoprolol, if not contraindicated.

DIGAMI

Diabetes Mellitus Insulin-Glucose Infusion in Acute Myocardial Infarction

(continued)

Results

Blood glucose decreased from 15.4±4.1 to 9.6±3.3 mmol/l in the infusion group over the first 24 h, and from 15.7±4.2 to 11.7±4.1 mmol/l among the control patients ($p<0.0001$). In-hospital mortality was 9.1% in the insulin vs 11.1% in the control group (p=NS). 1 year mortality was 18.6% vs 26.1%, respectively (relative risk reduction 29%, 95% CI 4%-51%, $p=0.0273$). The reduction in mortality was particularly evident in low-risk patients and with no previous insulin therapy (3 month mortality 6.5% in the insulin vs 13.5% in the control, relative risk reduction 52%, $p=0.046$; 1 year mortality 8.6% vs 18.0%, respectively, relative risk reduction 52%, $p=0.020$).

Conclusions

Insulin glucose infusion followed by a multidose insulin therapy improved 1 year survival in diabetic patients after acute myocardial infarction.

CRIS

Calcium antagonist Reinfarction Italian Study

Title	A controlled trial of verapamil in patients after acute myocardial infarction: results of the calcium antagonist reinfarction Italian study (CRIS).
Authors	Rengo F, Carbonin P, Pahor M, et al.
Reference	Am J Cardiol 1996;77:365-369.
Disease	Acute myocardial infarction
Purpose	To evaluate the effects of verapamil on total mortality, cardiac mortality, reinfarction, and recurrent angina after an acute myocardial infarction.
Design	Randomized, double blind, placebo controlled, multicenter.
Patients	1073 patients, age 30 to 75 years, who survived 5 days following an acute myocardial infarction. Patients with severe heart failure, Wolf-Parkinson-White syndrome, cardiac surgery, implanted pacemaker, right ventricular failure with pulmonary hypertension, concomitant severe disease, contraindication to verapamil, heart rate <50 beats/min, hypotension or hypertension, chronic therapy with β blockers or calcium channel blockers were excluded.
Follow-up	mean follow-up 23.5 months.
Treatment regimen	Seven to 21 days (mean 13.8 days) after myocardial infarction patients were randomized to placebo or verapamil retard 120 mgX3/d

CRIS

Calcium antagonist Reinfarction Italian Study

(continued)

Results Study medication was discontinued before completion of follow-up in 36.9% of the placebo group and 35.6% of the verapamil group. Intention to treat analysis revealed no difference in mortality (5.4% vs 5.6%), cardiac mortality (4.1% vs 4.0%;), and sudden death (1.8% vs 2.1%), in the placebo and verapamil group, respectively. There was a trend toward less reinfarction in the verapamil group (7.3% vs 9.0%; relative risk (RR) 0.81; 95% CI 0.53-1.24). Verapamil therapy was also associated with a non-significant reduction in the rates of first major event (death or reinfarction,9.0% vs 10.3%; RR 0.87; 95% CI 0.59-1.29), and first cardiac event (cardiac death, reinfarction, or hospital admission for chest pain, 15.4% vs 19.2%; RR 0.79; 95% CI 0.59-1.05). Less patients in the verapamil group developed angina (18.8% vs 24.3%; RR 0.8; 95% CI 0.5 to 0.9; $p<0.05$).

Conclusions Verapamil therapy following myocardial infarction was not associated with reduced mortality. However, it was associated with less angina and a trend toward less reinfarction.

EMIAT

The European Myocardial Infarct Amiodarone Trial

Title	Randomised trial of effect of amiodarone on mortality in patients with left-ventricular dysfunction after recent myocardial infarction: EMIAT
Author	Julian DG, Camm AJ, Frangin G, et al.
Reference	Lancet 1997;349:667-674.
Disease	Acute myocardial infarction.
Purpose	To assess the efficacy of amiodarone on reduction of mortality of patients with left ventricular dysfunction following myocardial infarction.
Design	Randomized, double blind, placebo controlled, multicenter.
Patients	1486 patients, 18-75 years old, 5-21 days (mean 15±3.9 days) after acute myocardial infarction with left ventricular ejection fraction <40%. Patients with contraindications to amiodarone, amiodarone therapy within 6 months, bradycardia <50 bpm, advanced atrioventricular block, hepatic disease, thyroid dysfunction, long QT syndrome, severe angina or heart failure, a likelihood of cardiac surgery, and those requiring active antiarrhythmic medications were excluded.
Follow-up	Clinical follow-up for 12 to 24 months (median 21 months). 24 h Holter ECG monitoring at baseline and after 2 weeks and 4 months.
Treatment regimen	Placebo or amiodarone (800 mg/d for 14 days, 400 mg/d for 14 weeks, and then 200 mg/d).
Additional therapy	β blockers and digoxin were permitted.

Results

743 patients were included in each group. All cause mortality was similar (103 patients in the amiodarone group vs 103 in the placebo patients; risk ratio (RR) 0.99; 95% CI 0.76-1.31; p=0.96). Cardiac mortality was comparable (85 vs 89 patients, respectively; RR 0.94; 95% CI 0.70-1.26; p=0.67). However, arrhythmic deaths (33 vs 50 patients; RR 0.65; 95% CI 0.42-1.00; p=0.05) and arrhythmic death and resuscitated cardiac arrest (42 vs 61 patients; RR 0.68; 95% CI 0.46-1.00; p=0.05) were less common in the amiodarone than the placebo group. However, death from reinfarction occurred in 10 amiodarone treated patients versus only 3 of the placebo treated patients. Non cardiac mortality occurred in 18 of the amiodarone vs 13% of the placebo patients (RR 1.37; 95% CI 0.67-2.79). In intention-to-treat analysis of the 548 patients with arrhythmias at baseline, there was no statistically significant difference between the amiodarone and placebo groups concerning arrhythmic death, but there was reduction in the occurrence of the combined end-point of arrhythmic deaths and resuscitated cardiac deaths in the amiodarone group (p=0.048). During the trial, 38.5% of the amiodarone vs 21.4% of the placebo group discontinued the study medication. Clinical hypothyroidism occurred in 1.5% vs 0% of the amiodarone and placebo groups, whereas hyperthyroidism in 1.6% vs 0.5%, respectively. Pulmonary disorders occurred in 5.2% vs 4.0%, respectively.

Conclusions

Amiodarone therapy in survivors of myocardial infarction with left ventricular dysfunction was not associated with reduction of total mortality or cardiac mortality during a median follow-up of 21 months. However, the reduction in arrhythmic death and the apparent lack of proarrhythmic effect support the use of amiodarone in patients with ischemic heart disease and left ventricular dysfunction for whom antiarrhythmic therapy is indicated.

CAMIAT

Canadian Amiodarone Myocardial Infarction Arrhythmia Trial

Title	Randomised trial of outcome after myocardial infarction in patients with frequent or repetitive ventricular premature depolarisations: CAMIAT
Authors	Cairns JA, Connolly SJ, Roberts R, et al.
Reference	Lancet 1997;349:675-682.
Disease	Acute myocardial infarction.
Purpose	To assess the efficacy of amiodarone on reduction of the risk of resuscitated ventricular fibrillation or arrhythmic death among patients with left ventricular dysfunction following myocardial infarction with frequent or repetitive ventricular premature depolarizations.
Design	Randomized, double blind, placebo controlled, multicenter.
Patients	1202 patients, >19 years old, 6-45 days after myocardial infarction, with a mean of 10 ventricular premature depolarizations per hour or more by 24 h ambulatory ECG monitoring, or ≥1 run of ventricular tachycardia. Patients with contraindications to amiodarone; bradycardia (<50 bpm); atrioventricular block; QTc >480 ms; peripheral neuropathy; liver disease; pulmonary fibrosis; asthma; thyroid disease; need for antiarrhythmic therapy; therapy with tricyclic antidepressants, phenytoin, or sotalol; severe congestive heart failure; hypotension or angina; and patients with life expectancy of <2 years were excluded.
Follow-up	Repeated 24 h ambulatory ECG monitoring at baseline, 4, 8, 12 and 16 months. Clinical follow-up for 1 to 2 years (mean 1.79±0.44 years).
Treatment regimen	Placebo or amiodarone (a loading dose of 10 mg/kg in two divided daily doses for 2 weeks, then 400 mg/d. Patients older than 75 years and those who weighed <60 kg received 300 mg/d). If arrhythmia suppression was detected, the dose was reduced to 200-300 mg/d at month 4 and to 200 mg/d for 5-7 days/week at month 8.

Results

There were 606 patients in the amiodarone group and 596 in the placebo group. 24 h ambulatory ECG monitoring at month 4 revealed arrhythmia suppression in 84% of the amiodarone group vs 35% of the placebo group, and at month 8 in 86% vs 39%, respectively. The mean percentage of study drug being taken at each follow-up visit was 75% and 78% in the amiodarone and placebo groups. Only 6% of the patients in each group took <50% of the study medication. 221 (36.4%) patients of the amiodarone group vs 152 (25.5%) of the placebo group discontinued taking study medication for reasons other than outcome events (p<0.0005). Adverse effects resulting in discontinuation of study medication occurred in 159 (26.2%) patients of the amiodarone vs 82 (13.7%) patients in the placebo group (p<0.0005). Hypothyroidism was found in 3.3% vs 0.2%, respectively (p<0.0005). Proarrhythmia (0.3% vs 3.0%; p=0.002) and ventricular tachyarrhythmia (0.7% vs 2.0%; p=0.004) occurred less often in the amiodarone treated patients. Efficacy analysis revealed that the estimated risk of resuscitated ventricular fibrillation or arrhythmic death at 24 months was 1.77% per year for the amiodarone vs 3.38% per year for the placebo groups (48.5% relative-risk reduction; 95% CI 4.5 to 72.2%; p=0.018). 37 vs 50 patients of the amiodarone and placebo group died (rate per year for all-cause mortality 4.36% vs 5.42%; relative-risk reduction 21.2%; 95% CI -20.6% to 48.5%; p=0.136). 30 vs 44 patients of the amiodarone and placebo group died from cardiac causes (rate per year 3.53% vs 4.77%; relative-risk reduction 27.4%; 95% CI -15.5% to 54.4%; p=0.087). Intention-to-treat analysis revealed reduction in the risk for resuscitated ventricular fibrillation or arrhythmic death (relative-risk reduction 38.2%; 95% CI -2.1% to 62.6%; p=0.029); arrhythmic death (29.3%; 95% CI -19.6% to 58.2%; p=0.097); cardiac mortality (22.0%; 95% CI -15.9% to 47.6%; p=0.108); and total mortality (18.3%; 95% CI -16.1% to 42.6%; p=0.129). The cumulative rates of non-arrhythmic death were comparable (5.8% in the amiodarone group vs 6.2% in the placebo group; p=0.70).

Conclusions

Amiodarone therapy in survivors of myocardial infarction with frequent or repetitive ventricular premature depolarizations was associated with reduction of ventricular fibrillation or arrhythmic death. No proarrhythmic effect was observed. However, adverse effects mandating discontinuation of amiodarone were relatively common.

2. Unstable Angina

RISC

Risk of myocardial infarction and death during treatment with low dose aspirin and intravenous heparin in men with unstable coronary artery disease

Title	Risk of myocardial infarction and death during treatment with low dose aspirin and intravenous heparin in men with unstable coronary artery disease.
Authors	The RISC Group.
Reference	Lancet 1990;336:827-830.
Disease	Unstable angina pectoris, non-Q-wave myocardial infarction.
Purpose	To evaluate the efficacy and safety of low dose aspirin and IV heparin therapy for patients with unstable angina or non-Q-wave infarction.
Design	Randomized, double blind, placebo controlled, 2X2 factorial, multicenter.
Patients	796 men, <70 years old, with unstable angina or non-Q-wave infarction. Patients with left ventricular dysfunction from previous infarction or valvular disease, previous coronary bypass grafting surgery, permanent pacemaker, left bundle branch block, or inability to complete exercise test were excluded.
Follow-up	>3 months.
Treatment regimen	Randomization within 72 h after admission to: oral aspirin 75 mg/d or placebo for 1 year, and to IV placebo or heparin 10,000 U X4/d as a bolus for the first day and 7,500 U X4/d for 4 more days.
Additional therapy	No drug containing aspirin, NSAID, or anticoagulant was permitted. If not contraindicated, metoprolol 100-200 mg/d. Nitrates and calcium channel blockers were permitted.

RISC

Risk of myocardial infarction and death during treatment with low dose aspirin and intravenous heparin in men with unstable coronary artery disease

(continued)

Results

Myocardial infarction or death occurred in 5.8% vs 2.5% of the oral placebo and aspirin groups respectively after 5 days (RR 0.43, 95% CI 0.21-0.91, p=0.033). After 30 days the incidence was 13.4% vs 4.3% (RR 0.31, 95% CI 0.18-0.53, p<0.0001), while after 90 days it was 17.1% vs 6.5% (RR 0.36, 95% CI 0.23-0.57, p<0.0001), respectively. Treatment with intermittent bolus injections of heparin did not alter the rates of myocardial infarction or death, although the group treated with aspirin and heparin had the lowest number of events during the initial 5 days. Treatment was associated with few side effects and was well tolerated.

Conclusions

Low dose aspirin, but not intermittent bolus injections of heparin, reduced mortality and myocardial infarction rates in patients with unstable angina or non-Q-wave infarction.

UNASEM

Unstable Angina Study using Eminase

Title	Thrombolysis in patients with unstable angina improves the angiographic but not the clinical outcome. Results of UNASEM, a multicenter, randomized, placebo-controlled, clinical trial with anistreplase.
Authors	Bär FW, Verheugt FW, Col J, et al.
Reference	Circulation 1992;86:131-137.
Disease	Unstable angina.
Purpose	To evaluate the role of thrombolytic therapy in unstable angina.
Design	Randomized, double blind, placebo controlled, multicenter.
Patients	126 patients, age 30-70 years, with unstable angina with electrocardiographic evidence of ischemia. Patients with previous infarction, angioplasty, cardiac surgery, cardiac pacemaker, intraventricular conduction abnormalities, valvular heart disease, hypertension, cardiomyopathy, heart failure, renal failure, anticoagulant therapy, or contraindication to thrombolysis were excluded. Patients with left main stenosis ≥70% or <50% stenosis of the coronary arteries were excluded.
Follow-up	Coronary angiography before randomization and after 12-28 h.
Treatment regimen	IV injection of 30 U anistreplase (APSAC) or placebo over 5 min after the first cardiac catheterization.

UNASEM

Unstable Angina Study using Eminase

(continued)

Additional therapy

IV nitroglycerin started before angiography. IV heparin 5,000 U bolus followed by infusion at a rate of 1,000 U/h. ß blockers or calcium blockers were given routinely. Aspirin was given after the second angiogram. Angioplasty was recommended only for recurrent angina in spite of medical therapy.

Results

Anistreplase compared to placebo was associated with decrease in diameter stenosis between the baseline to follow-up angiography (11% change (70% to 59%) vs 3% change (66% to 63%), p=0.008). However, clinical outcome was not different. Bleeding complications were higher in the anistreplase group (32% vs 11%, p=0.001).

Conclusions

Anistreplase infusion was associated with angiographic, but not clinical improvement. Moreover, it was associated with excess of bleeding.

TIMI IIIA

Thrombolysis in Myocardial Ischemia Trial IIIA

Title	Early effects of tissue-type plasminogen activator added to conventional therapy on the culprit coronary lesion in patients presenting with ischemic cardiac pain at rest. Results of the Thrombolysis in Myocardial Ischemia (TIMI IIIA) Trial.
Authors	The TIMI IIIA Investigators.
Reference	Circulation 1993;87:38-52.
Disease	Unstable angina, non-Q wave myocardial infarction.
Purpose	To assess the early effects of t-PA on the culprit coronary lesion in patients with unstable angina or non-Q wave myocardial infarction.
Design	Randomized, placebo controlled, multicenter.
Patients	306 patients age 22-75 years with ≥5 min but ≤6 h of chest pain occurring at rest accompanied by ECG changes or documented coronary artery disease.
Follow-up	Coronary angiography at baseline and after 18-48 h.
Treatment regimen	Tissue plasminogen activator (t-PA) at a total dose of 0.8 mg/kg (maximum total dose 80 mg) or placebo infusion over 90 min (1/3 of the total dose was given as a bolus).
Additional therapy	Bed rest, oxygen, nitrates, calcium antagonists, and/or ß blockers, heparin 5000 U bolus and infusion for 18-48 h.

Results

Reduction of stenosis by ≥20% or improvement of TIMI flow by 2 grades was seen in 15% and 5% of the culprit lesions in the t-PA and placebo-treated patients (p=0.003). Substantial improvement was seen more often with t-PA (36%) than placebo (15%) among lesions containing thrombus (p<0.01), and among patients with non-Q wave infarction (33% versus 8%, respectively, p<0.005). By multivariate analysis, the adjusted p value for substantial improvement of the culprit lesion by t-PA was 0.01

Conclusions

Angiographic improvement of the severity of the culprit lesion after conventional therapy with and without additional t-PA was only modest. However, substantial improvement of the culprit lesions was seen more frequently with t-PA than placebo, especially in two subgroups: those with apparent thrombus and those with non-Q wave infarction.

TIMI IIIB

Thrombolysis in Myocardial Ischemia Trial IIIB

Title	Effects of tissue plasminogen activator and a comparison of early invasive and conservative strategies in unstable angina and non-Q-wave myocardial infarction. Results of the TIMI IIIB Trial.
Authors	The TIMI IIIB Investigators.
Reference	Circulation 1994;89:1545-1556.
Disease	Unstable angina, non-Q wave myocardial infarction.
Purpose	To assess the early effects of t-PA and of an early invasive strategy on clinical outcome of patients with unstable angina or non-Q wave myocardial infarction.
Design	Randomized, placebo controlled, multicenter.
Patients	1473 patients age 22-79 years with ≥5 min but ≤6 h of chest pain occurring at rest accompanied by ECG changes or documented coronary artery disease.
Follow-up	24-h Holter monitoring that began 60-120 h after randomization. Predischarge thallium scintigraphy. Clinical evaluation and exercise tolerance test at 6 weeks.
Treatment regimen	Tissue plasminogen activator (t-PA) at a total dose of 0.8 mg/kg (maximum total dose 80 mg) or placebo infusion over 90 min (1/3 of the total dose was given as a bolus). Patients were also randomized to early invasive and early conservative strategies. In the early invasive group patients underwent coronary angiography 18-48 h after randomization and followed by revascularization if suitable. In the conservative arm patients were referred to coronary angiography only after failure of initial therapy.

TIMI IIIB

Thrombolysis in Myocardial Ischemia Trial IIIB

(continued)

Additional therapy

Bed rest, oxygen, a long acting nitrate, ß blockers, calcium antagonists, and heparin 5000 U bolus and infusion for 18-48 h. Aspirin 325 mg/d was began on the second day and continued for 1 year.

Results

The primary end point of death, myocardial infarction, or failure of initial therapy at 6 weeks occurred in 54.2% and 55.5% of the t-PA and placebo treated groups. Acute myocardial infarction was more prevalent in the t-PA (7.4%) than placebo treated patients (4.9%, p=0.04). Intracranial hemorrhage occurred in 0.55% and 0 of the t-PA and placebo groups (p=0.06).
The primary end point for comparison between the early invasive and conservative group (death, myocardial infarction, or an unsatisfactory symptom-limited exercise test at 6 weeks) occurred in 18.1% and 16.2% of the early conservative and early invasive strategies, respectively (p=NS). However, the initial hospitalization was shorter and the incidence of rehospitalization was lower in the early invasive treated patients.

Conclusions

The addition of t-PA was not beneficial and may even be harmful. There was no difference in the primary end points between the early invasive and conservative strategies, although the former resulted in a shorter hospitalization and lower rate of readmission.

TAUSA

Thrombolysis and Angioplasty in Unstable Angina

Title	a. Adjunctive thrombolytic therapy during angioplasty for ischemic rest angina: results of the TAUSA Trial. b. Angioplasty of complex lesions in ischemic rest angina: results of the Thrombolysis and Angioplasty in Unstable Angina (TAUSA) Trial.
Authors	a. Ambrose JA, Almeida OD, Sharma S, et al. b. Mehran R, Ambrose JA, Bongu RM, et al.
Reference	a. Circulation 1994;90:69-77. b. J Am Coll Cardiol 1995;26:961-966.
Disease	Coronary artery disease, unstable angina.
Purpose	To assess the role of prophylactic intracoronary thrombolytic therapy during coronary angioplasty in unstable angina.
Design	Randomized, double blind, placebo controlled, multicenter.
Patients	469 patients with unstable angina with ischemic rest pain or non-Q wave infarction <7 d before angioplasty, or recurrent rest pain within 7 days <30 d after myocardial infarction. All patients had ≥70 % stenosis of a native artery or vein graft that was suitable for angioplasty. Patients >80 years old, severe hypertension, prior stroke or contraindications to thrombolytic therapy were excluded.
Follow-up	Angiography 15 min after angioplasty. In hospital clinical follow-up.
Treatment regimen	Phase I: Urokinase 150,000 U or placebo over 3 min (Phase I) or 250,000 U or placebo over 10-15 min (Phase II), before wire placement. Additional 100,000 U (Phase I) or 250,000 U (Phase II) or placebo 1 min post angioplasty.

TAUSA

Thrombolysis and Angioplasty in Unstable Angina

(continued)

Additional therapy	Aspirin 80-325 mg and IV heparin 10,000 U before procedure. 75 μg intracoronary nitroglycerin before wire placement. IV heparin infusion overnight.
Results	a. 257 and 212 patients were included in phase I and II, respectively. Angioplasty was successful in 97% and 94% of the placebo and urokinase groups (p=NS). Definite filling defects were present at 15 min in 18.0% vs 13.8% of the placebo and urokinase patients (p=NS). Acute closure was more common with urokinase (10.2%) than placebo (4.3%, p<0.02). These differences were more pronounced in phase II (8.7% vs 1.9%, p=0.031) than in phase I. There was no difference in detection of coronary dissection between the groups. Emergency bypass surgery (5.2% vs 2.1%, p=0.09) and post procedure ischemia (9.9% vs 3.4%, p=0.005) were more common in the urokinase group, however, there was no difference in the occurrence of myocardial infarction. Bleeding complications were reported in 12.9% and 8.9% of the urokinase and placebo groups (p=NS). b. Complex lesions were associated with higher abrupt closure than simple lesions (10.6% vs 3.3%, p<0.003), and higher recurrent angina. Abrupt closure of the complex lesions was more common in the urokinase group (15.0% vs 5.9%, p<0.03).
Conclusions	Prophylactic urokinase intracoronary administration was associated with adverse angiographic and clinical outcome in patients with unstable angina undergoing coronary angioplasty.

ATACS

Antithrombotic Therapy in Acute Coronary Syndromes

Title Combination antithrombotic therapy in unstable rest angina and non-Q-wave infarction in nonprior aspirin users. Primary end points analysis from the ATACS trial.

Authors Cohen M, Adams PC, Parry G, et al.

Reference Circulation 1994;89:81-88.

Disease Unstable angina, non Q wave myocardial infarction.

Purpose To compare the efficacy of combination of aspirin + anticoagulation vs aspirin alone in patients with rest unstable angina or non-Q-wave infarction.

Design Randomized, open label, multicenter.

Patients 214 patients, >21 years of age, with unstable rest angina or non Q wave infarction. Patients that received ≥150 mg aspirin within 3 d of randomization were excluded.

Follow-up 12 weeks.

Treatment regimen Aspirin 162.5 mg/d or aspirin 162.5 mg/d +heparin 100 U/kg IV bolus and then continuous infusion of heparin for 3-4 days. Warfarin was started on the 2nd-3rd day, if coronary angiography did not appear imminent. Heparin was discontinued after INR reached 2.0-3.0.

Additional therapy Antianginal therapy: low risk patients received metoprolol and oral isosorbide dinitrate; high risk patients received additional nifedipine. If ß blockers were contraindicated, diltiazem was given instead of metoprolol. Patients already on ß blockers, received maximal dose of ß blockers + nifedipine.

ATACS

Antithrombotic Therapy in Acute Coronary Syndromes

(continued)

Results

Trial therapy was begun by 9.5±8.8 h of qualifying pain. By intention to treat analysis, after 14 days 27% of the aspirin vs 10% of the aspirin+anticoagulation experienced death, recurrent angina or infarction (adjusted p=0.004). After 12 weeks 28% of the aspirin vs 19% of the aspirin+anticoagulation experienced death, recurrent angina or infarction (adjusted p=0.09). Major bleeding complications occurred in 0 and 2.9%, respectively, while minor bleeding or medication intolerance was found in 2.8% and 6.7%, respectively. Withdrawal from the study or occurrence of a secondary end point (major bleeding or coronary revascularization) occurred in 31% and 45%, respectively.

Conclusions

Combination of anticoagulation therapy and aspirin, compared with aspirin alone, significantly reduced recurrent ischemic events in the early phase of unstable angina or non-Q wave infarction.

Title	Recombinant hirudin for unstable unstable angina pectoris. A multicenter, randomized angiographic trial.
Authors	Topol EJ, Fuster V, Harrington RA, et al.
Reference	Circulation 1994;89:1557-1566.
Disease	Unstable angina pectoris.
Purpose	To compare the efficacy of hirudin and heparin in preventing accumulation of coronary artery thrombus in patients with unstable angina.
Design	Randomized, open label, comparing 2 regimens of heparin and 4 regimens of hirudin in multifactorial fashion, multicenter.
Patients	166 patients, ≤75 years of age, with ≥5 min of rest ischemic pain within 48 h, and ≥60% stenosis of a major epicardial coronary artery or vein graft interpreted as having an intraluminal thrombus. Patients with renal failure, hemodynamic instability, previous stroke, or history of significant bleeding were excluded.
Follow-up	Coronary angiography at baseline and after 72-120 h. Clinical follow-up for 30 days.
Treatment regimen	1. Hirudin 0.15 mg/kg bolus, 0.05 mg/kg/h infusion. 2. Hirudin 0.30 mg/kg bolus, 0.1 mg/kg/h infusion. 3. Hirudin 0.60 mg/kg bolus, 0.2 mg/kg/h infusion. 4. Hirudin 0.90 mg/kg bolus, 0.3 mg/kg/h infusion. 5. Hirudin 0.60 mg/kg bolus, 0.3 mg/kg/h infusion. 6. Hirudin 0.60 mg/kg bolus, 0.3 mg/kg/h infusion. In all regimens:heparin 5000 U bolus, 1000 U/h infusion. PTT was adjusted to 65-90 s in regimens 1-5, and to 90-110 s in regimen 6. Infusion was continued for 3-5 days.

(continued)

Additional therapy	Aspirin 160-325 mg/d. ß blockers, calcium channel blockers, and long acting nitrate. Coronary revascularization was discouraged until completion of the second angiogram.
Results	Hirudin led to a dose-dependent prolongation of the PTT that appeared to plateau at the 0.2 mg/kg/h infusion rate. 16% of the heparin and 71% of the hirudin treated patients had their aPTT within the therapeutic range ($p<0.001$). The hirudin treated patients showed better improvement in minimal cross sectional area of the culprit lesion (0.29 vs 0.10 mm^2, $p=0.028$), minimal luminal diameter (0.18 vs 0.03 mm, $p=0.029$), and % diameter stenosis (-5.19% vs -2.11%, $p=0.071$). There was no difference in any of the clinical events at 30 days between heparin and hirudin. There was no major adverse effects associated with hirudin.
Conclusions	Recombinant hirudin in patients with unstable angina improved the angiographic results, but not the clinical outcome.

TIMI-7

Thrombin Inhibition in Myocardial Ischemia 7

Title	Hirulog in the treatment of unstable angina. Results of the thrombin inhibition in myocardial ischemia (TIMI) 7 trial.
Authors	Fuchs J, Cannon CP, and the TIMI 7 Investigators.
Reference	Circulation 1995;92:727-733.
Disease	Unstable angina.
Purpose	To assess whether a dose response existed in the efficacy of hirulog used in conjunction with aspirin in unstable angina.
Design	randomized, double blind, multicenter.
Patients	401 patients, age 21-75 years, with unstable angina (ischemic rest pain of 5-60 min) within 24 h of randomization, >24 h after myocardial infarction (if present).
Follow-up	6 weeks.
Treatment regimen	One of 4 doses of hirulog infusion for 72 h: 0.02, 0.25, 0.50, and 1.0 mg/kg/h.
Additional therapy	Aspirin 325 mg/d. No restriction on conventional therapy, excluding heparin during hirulog infusion.

Results

There was no difference among the groups in the primary end point (death, myocardial infarction, rapid clinical deterioration, or recurrent ischemia with ECG changes) at 72 h (primary end point occurred in 8.1%, 6.2%, 11.4%, and 6.2% of the patients in the 4 groups, respectively, p=0.56). Primary end points occurred in 15.0%, 7.4%, 14.8%, and 12.3% of the patients respectively at discharge (p=0.38). However, death or recurrent infarction at discharge occurred in 10% of the 0.02 mg/kg/h group vs 3.2% of the patients assigned to the 3 other groups (p=0.008). After 6 weeks end point occurred in 12.5% of the lower dose vs 5.2% of the upper three doses (p=0.009). Only 0.5% (2 patients) experienced a major bleeding attributed to hirulog.

Conclusions

Hirulog in conjunction with aspirin is a safe and promising therapy for unstable angina.

A Comparison of Hirudin with Heparin in the Prevention of Restenosis after Coronary Angioplasty

Title	A comparison of hirudin with heparin in the prevention of restenosis after coronary angioplasty.
Authors	Serruys PW, Herrman JP, Simon R, et al.
Reference	N Engl J Med 1995;333:757-763.
Disease	Coronary artery disease, unstable angina.
Purpose	To compare the efficacy of two regimens of recombinant hirudin with heparin in preventing restenosis following coronary angioplasty.
Design	Randomized, double blind, multicenter.
Patients	1141 patients with unstable angina with ≥1 lesion suitable for coronary angioplasty.
Follow-up	30 week clinical follow-up, coronary angiography after 26 weeks.
Treatment regimen	1. Recombinant hirudin IV 40 mg bolus followed by infusion of 0.2 mg/kg/h for 24 h, and then placebo X2/d SC for 3 days. 2. Recombinant hirudin IV 40 mg bolus followed by infusion of 0.2 mg/kg/h for 24 h, and then 40 mg X2/d SC for 3 days. 3. Heparin 10,000 U bolus followed by infusion of 15 U/kg/h for 24 h, and then placebo X2/d SC for 3 days.
Additional therapy	Aspirin 100-500 mg/d for ≥14 days.

A Comparison of Hirudin with Heparin in the Prevention of Restenosis after Coronary Angioplasty

(continued)

Results At 30 weeks, event-free survival was 67.3%, 63.5%, and 68.0% for the heparin, hirudin IV, and hirudin IV+SC (p=0.61). However, early cardiac events (within 96 h) were reduced by hirudin (occurrence in 11.0%, 7.9%, and 5.6%, respectively, combined relative risk with hirudin vs heparin 0.61, 95% CI 0.41-0.90, p=0.023). In patients with severe unstable angina (Braunwald class III) the 96 h event rates were 21.6%, 5.3%, and 12.3% (combined relative risk 0.41, 95% CI 0.21-0.78, p=0.006). The minimal luminal diameter on the follow-up angiography was 1.54, 1.47, and 1.56 mm, respectively (p=0.08).

Conclusions Although hirudin reduced the occurrence of early complications, long-term results were the same as with heparin.

HASI

Hirulog Angioplasty Study Investigators

Title	Treatment with bivaliridun (hirulog) as compared with heparin during coronary angioplasty for unstable or postinfarction angina.
Authors	Bittl JA, Strony J, Brinker JA, et al.
Reference	N Engl J Med 1995;333:764-769.
Disease	Unstable angina
Purpose	To compare the efficacy of hirulog and heparin as an adjunctive therapy after angioplasty for unstable or postinfarction angina.
Design	Randomized, double blind, multicenter.
Patients	4098 patients, >21 years old, with unstable or postinfarction angina <2 week after infarction.
Follow-up	In-hospital, 3 and 6 months clinical course.
Treatment regimen	1. Hirulog: 1.0 mg/kg bolus before angioplasty, followed by 4 h infusion at a rate of 2.5 mg/kg/h, and a 14-20 h infusion at a rate of 0.2 mg/kg/h. 2. Heparin: IV bolus 175 U/kg followed by infusion at a rate of 15 U/kg/h for 18-24 h.
Additional therapy	Aspirin 300-325 mg/d.

HASI

Hirulog Angioplasty Study Investigators

(continued)

Results

In the total population the occurrence of the primary end point (death, myocardial infarction, abrupt closure, or rapid clinical deterioration requiring coronary bypass surgery, intra-aortic balloon counterpulsation, or repeated angioplasty) were similar between the hirulog (11.4%) and heparin (12.2%). However, hirulog resulted in lower incidence of major bleeding (3.8% vs 9.8%, $p<0.001$). In the subpopulation of postinfarction angina, hirulog resulted in a lower incidence of the in-hospital primary end points (9.1% vs 14.2%, $p=0.04$), lower incidence of myocardial infarction (2.0% vs 5.1%, $p=0.04$) and a lower incidence of bleeding (3.0% vs 11.1%, $p<0.001$). However, the cumulative rate of death, myocardial infarction, and repeated revascularization in the postinfarction angina patients during the 6 months follow-up were similar (20.5% vs 25.1%, $p=0.17$).

Conclusions

Hirulog (bivalirudin) was as effective as high dose heparin in preventing the ischemic complications following angioplasty for unstable angina. It was better than heparin in reducing the immediate complications in patients with postinfarction angina. Hirulog was associated with a lower incidence of bleeding.

FRISC

Fragmin During Instability in Coronary Artery Disease Study

Title	Low-molecular-weight heparin during instability in coronary artery disease.
Authors	Fragmin during Instability in Coronary Artery Disease (FRISC) Study Group.
Reference	Lancet 1996;347:561-568.
Disease	Unstable angina, non-Q-wave infarction.
Purpose	To assess the efficacy of subcutaneous low-molecular-weight heparin, in combination with aspirin and antianginal medications, to prevent new cardiac events in patients with unstable angina.
Design	Randomized, double blind, placebo controlled, multicenter.
Patients	1506 patients, >40 years old, with unstable angina (<72 h from the last episode of chest pain). Premenopausal women, patients with an increased risk of bleeding, current treatment with anticoagulants, or coronary revascularization within 3 months were excluded.
Follow-up	150 days clinical follow-up. Predischarge and 40-50 day exercise test.
Treatment regimen	Placebo or dalteparin sodium 120 U/kg (maximum 10,000 U)X2/d SC for 6 days, and then 7,500 U X1/d for the next 35-45 days.
Additional therapy	Aspirin 75 mg/d (initial dose 300 mg), ß blockers, nitrates and calcium channel blockers.

FRISC

Fragmin During Instability in Coronary Artery Disease Study

(continued)

Results

6 day mortality or development of new myocardial infarction was 4.8% in the placebo and 1.8% in the dalteparin group (RR 0.37, 95% CI 0.20-0.68, p=0.001). 1.2% vs 0.4%, respectively needed revascularization (RR 0.33, 95% CI 0.10-1.10, p=0.07), while 7.7% vs 3.8% needed intravenous heparin (RR 0.49, 95% CI 0.32-0.75, p=0.001). After 40 days the rate of death, myocardial infarction, revascularization or the need for IV heparin was 25.7% in the placebo vs 20.5% in the dalteparin group (RR 0.79, 95% CI 0.66-0.95, p=0.011). There was an increased event rate during the first few days after the change of the dose in the dalteparin group, especially in smokers. There was no difference in the rates of end points after 150 d. The regimen was relatively safe with rare side effects, and compliance was good.

Conclusions

Long term dalteparin and aspirin therapy is safe and effective in patients with unstable angina.

The Canadian Lamifiban Study

Title
Platelet membrane receptor glycoprotein IIb/IIIa antagonism in unstable angina. The Canadian Lamifiban study.

Authors
Thèroux P, Kouz S, Roy L, et al.

Reference
Circulation 1996;94:899-905.

Disease
Coronary artery disease, unstable angina.

Purpose
To assess the clinical benefit of GP IIb/IIIa inhibition by Lamifiban in patients with unstable angina.

Design
Randomized, double blind, placebo-controlled, dose-ranging multicenter.

Patients
365 patients, <75 years old, with unstable angina or myocardial infarction without ST segment elevation. Patients with identifiable precipitating secondary factors, or <6 months after PTCA or <2 months after coronary artery bypass surgery were excluded. Additional exclusion criteria were previous stroke, high risk for bleeding, uncontrolled hypertension, congestive heart failure or shock, thrombocytopenia, use of oral anticoagulants, concomitant life threatening disease, and left bundle branch block.

Follow-up
One month.

Treatment regimen
Patients were randomized to one of five parallel arms: placebo and 4 doses of lamifiban. All arms included an IV bolus followed by an infusion for 72-120 hours. The bolus plus infusion doses were 1) 150 μg + 1μg/min; 2) 300 μg + 2 μg/kg; 3) 600 μg + 4 μg/min; and 4) 750 μg + 5 μg/min. Three patients were randomized to lamifiban 600 μg bolus + 4 μg/min or to placebo for one patient in each of the other three groups.

Additional therapy

Aspirin 325 mg/d. Heparin was permitted. The use of nitrates, ß blockers, and/or calcium channel blockers was recommended.

Results

During the infusion period the lamifiban-treated patients (all doses) had lower rate of primary end-point (death, myocardial infarction, or the need for an urgent revascularization) from 8.1% in the placebo group to 3.3% (odds ratio 0.39; 95% CI 0.15 to 0.99; p=0.04). The rates were 2.5%, 4.9%, 3.3%, and 2.4%, respectively for the four lamifiban dosage groups. The highest dose (5 μg/min) had an additional benefit on recurrent ischemia over the three other lower doses (odds ratio compared with placebo 0.32; 95% CI 0.12 to 0.89; p=0.02). At one month, mortality was 4.1% in the placebo vs 1.2% in the lamifiban-treated patients. Death or myocardial infarction occurred in 8.1% of the placebo, 6.2% of the 2 lower lamifiban doses, and 2.5% of the patients treated with the higher doses of lamifiban. The odds ratio with the two high doses compared with placebo was 0.29 (95% CI 0.09 to 0.94; p=0.03). Lamifiban inhibited platelet aggregation in a dose-dependent fashion. Bleeding was more frequent with lamifiban than placebo (11.1% vs 1.6% of minor bleeding (p=0.002), and 2.9% vs 0.8% of minor bleeding (p=NS)). Concomitant heparin therapy increased significantly the bleeding risk.

Conclusions

3 to 5 days lamifiban therapy reduced the rate of mortality, myocardial infarction or the need for revascularization during the infusion period and at 1 month in patients with unstable angina

3. Stable Angina Pectoris and Silent Ischemia-Medical Therapy

ASIST

Atenolol Silent Ischemia Study

Title	Effects of treatment on outcome in mildly symptomatic patients with ischemia during daily life: the Atenolol Silent Ischemia Study (ASIST).
Authors	Pepine CJ, Cohn PF, Deedwania PC, et al.
Reference	Circulation 1994;90:762-768.
Disease	Coronary artery disease, silent myocardial ischemia
Purpose	To assess whether atenolol therapy will decrease adverse outcome events in mildly symptomatic patients with coronary artery disease.
Design	Randomized, double-blind, placebo controlled, multicenter.
Patients	306 patients with >50% stenosis of a major coronary artery, or previous myocardial infarction and transient ischemia documented by exercise ECG. Only patients with Canadian Cardiovascular Society class I or II, and without an abnormal ECG that could interfere with ambulatory ECG ST segment monitoring were included. Patients with unstable angina, myocardial infarction, or coronary revascularization within 3 month were excluded. Patients with contraindications to ß-blockers or with a need for antianginal medications other than nitrates, and patients with heart failure were excluded. The atenolol group included 152 patients and the placebo 154 patients.
Follow-up	1 year.
Treatment regimen	Atenolol (100 mg/d, in cases where adverse effects occurred, the dose was lowered to 50 mg/d) or placebo.

ASIST

Atenolol Silent Ischemia Study

(continued)

Results

After 4 weeks of therapy, the number (3.6±4.2 versus 1.7±4.6 episodes, $p<0.001$) and mean duration (30.0±3.3 versus 16.4±6.7 minutes, $p<0.001$) of ischemic episodes detected by 48 hours of ambulatory ECG monitoring were reduced in the atenolol treated patients, compared to baseline recording, but not in the placebo group. After one year less patients in the atenolol group experienced death, VT/VF, myocardial infarction, hospitalization, aggravation of angina, or revascularization (11% versus 25%; relative risk 44%; 95% CI 26-75%; $p=0.001$). The atenolol treated patients had a longer time to first event (120 versus 79 days; $p<0.001$). The most significant predictor of event-free survival in univariate and multivariate analysis was absence of ischemia on ambulatory ECG monitoring at 4 weeks. Side effects were comparable in both groups.

Conclusions

Treatment of asymptomatic or mildly symptomatic patients with coronary artery disease with atenolol reduced number and duration of ischemic episodes at 4 weeks and the risk for adverse events at one year.

CAPE

Circadian Anti-Ischemia Program in Europe

Title	Amlodipine reduces transient myocardial ischemia in patients with coronary artery disease: double-blind circadian anti-ischemia program in Europe (CAPE Trial).
Authors	Deanfield JE, Detry J-M RG, Lichtlen PR. et al.
Reference	J Am Coll Cardiol 1994;24:1460-1467.
Disease	Coronary artery disease, angina pectoris.
Purpose	To evaluate the effect of once-daily amlodipine on the circadian pattern of myocardial ischemia in patients with stable angina pectoris.
Design	Randomized, double blind, placebo controlled, multicenter.
Patients	315 males, age 35-80 years, with stable angina with ≥3 attacks/week. Patients with heart failure, uncontrolled arrhythmias, bradycardia, hypertension or hypotension, chronic therapy with calcium channel blockers, and ECG features that interfere with interpretation of ST segment changes were excluded. All patients had ≥4 ischemic episodes or ≥20 min of ST depression over 48 h ambulatory ECG monitoring.
Follow-up	Clinical follow-up and 48 h ambulatory monitoring at 8 weeks of phase II.
Treatment regimen	Phase I: 2 weeks of single blind placebo run-in period. Phase II: randomization to amlodipine (started at 5 mg/d and increased to 10 mg/d) or placebo treatment for 8 weeks.
Additional therapy	Patients were instructed to maintain on stable doses of all concomitant cardiovascular medications. Nitroglycerin tablets were provided.

CAPE

Circadian Anti-Ischemia Program in Europe

(continued)

Results Only 250 patients were fully evaluated for ambulatory ECG analysis. Amlodipine therapy resulted in greater reduction of the frequency of ST depression episodes (median reduction 60.0% vs 43.8%, p=0.025), ST segment integral (mm-min of ST depression)(median reduction 61.6% vs 49.5%, p=0.042), and total duration of ST depression (56% vs 49.5%, p=0.066) than placebo. The intrinsic circadian pattern of ischemia was maintained in both groups. Patients' diaries showed a significant reduction of anginal pain (70% vs 44%, p=0.0001), and in nitroglycerin consumption (67% vs 22%, p=0.0006) with amlodipine vs placebo. Adverse effects occurred in 17.3% of the amlodipine vs 13.3% of the placebo (p=0.422), discontinuation due to adverse events were 2.0% vs 4.4%, respectively (p=0.291).

Conclusions Once-daily amlodipine, in addition to regular anti-anginal therapy, reduced both symptomatic and asymptomatic ischemic episodes in patients with chronic stable angina.

ACIP

Asymptomatic Cardiac Ischemia Pilot Study

Title

a. The asymptomatic cardiac ischemia pilot (ACIP) study: design of a randomized clinical trial, baseline data and implications for a long-term outcome trial.
b. Effects of treatment strategies to suppress ischemia in patients with coronary artery disease: 12-week results of the asymptomatic cardiac ischemia pilot (ACIP) study.
c. Asymptomatic cardiac ischemia pilot (ACIP) study: impact of anti-ischemia therapy on 12-week rest electrocardiogram and exercise test outcomes.
d. Asymptomatic cardiac ischemia pilot (ACIP) study. Improvement of cardiac ischemia at 1 year after PTCA and CABG.

Authors

a. Pepine CJ, Geller NL, Knatterud GL, et al.
b. Knatterud GL, Bourassa MG, Pepine CJ, et al.
c. Chaitman BR, Stone PH, Knatterud GL, et al.
d. Bourassa MG, Knatterud GL, Pepine CJ, et al.

Reference

a. J Am Coll Cardiol 1994;24:1-10.
b. J Am Coll Cardiol 1994;24:11-20.
c. J Am Coll Cardiol 1995;26:585-593.
d. Circulation 1995;92:II-1-II-7.

Disease

Coronary artery disease.

Purpose

To compare three strategies of therapy (angina-guided medical therapy, ischemia-guided medical therapy, and coronary revascularization) in reduction of myocardial ischemia at exercise testing after 12 weeks of therapy.

Design

Randomized, open label, multicenter.

Patients

a+b. 618 patients, c+d. 558 patients with obstructive coronary artery disease suitable for revascularization, ≥1 episode of ischemia on 48 h ambulatory ECG monitoring, or evidence of ischemia on exercise test.

Follow-up	12 week repeated exercise test. 1 year clinical follow-up.
Treatment regimen	1. Angina guided medical therapy. 2. Angina + ambulatory ECG monitoring-guided medical therapy. 3. Coronary revascularization. The medical therapy included randomization to either atenolol or diltiazem as the first drug, and addition of nifedipine to atenolol and isosorbide dinitrate to diltiazem.
Results	a+b. Ambulatory ECG ischemia was no longer present at 12 week in 39%, 41%, and 55% of the angina-guided, ischemia-guided, and revascularization strategies. All strategies reduced the median number of episode and total duration of ST depression. Revascularization was the most effective strategy ($p<0.001$, and $p=0.01$ for the number of episodes and total duration, respectively). More patients were ischemia free in the atenolol + nifedipine (47%) than diltiazem + nitrates (32%, $p=0.03$). c. Peak exercise time was increased by 0.5, 0.7, and 1.6 min in the angina-guided, ischemia-guided, and revascularization strategies from baseline to 12 weeks ($p<0.001$). The sum of exercise induced ST depression was similar at baseline. However, at 12 weeks ST depression during exercise was 7.4±5.7, 6.8±5.3, and 5.6±5.6 mm, ($p=0.02$). d. At 12 weeks, ischemia on the ambulatory ECG monitoring was suppressed in 70% of the 78 CABG patients and in 46% of the 92 PTCA patients ($p=0.002$). Myocardial infarction or repeated revascularization occurred in 1 vs 7 of the CABG and PTCA patients ($p<0.001$).
Conclusions	Coronary revascularization significantly reduced the duration of silent ischemia on ambulatory ECG monitoring and the extent and frequency of exercise induced ischemia compared to the medical strategies.

TIBBS

Total Ischemic Burden Bisoprolol Study

Title	Medical treatment to reduce total ischemic burden: total ischemic burden bisoprolol study (TIBBS), a multicenter trial comparing bisoprolol and nifedipine.
Authors	von Arnim T, for the TIBBS Investigators.
Reference	J Am Coll Cardiol 1995;25:231-238.
Disease	Coronary artery disease, stable angina pectoris.
Purpose	To compare the effects of bisoprolol and nifedipine on transient myocardial ischemia in patients with stable angina.
Design	Randomized, double blind, multicenter.
Patients	330 patients with stable angina pectoris, positive exercise test with ST depression, and ≥2 episodes of transient myocardial ischemia on 48 h ambulatory ECG monitoring. Patients with unstable angina, myocardial infarction within 3 months, bradycardia <50 bpm, AV block, or hypotension were excluded.
Follow-up	Exercise test and ambulatory ECG monitoring during the placebo phase, after 4 weeks of the first dose period and after 8 weeks (double dose period).
Treatment regimen	10-day placebo phase, and then randomization to either bisoprolol 10 mg/d or nifedipine slow release 20 mg X2/d for 4 weeks, and then the doses were doubled for an additional 4 weeks.
Additional therapy	Long acting nitrates, ß blockers, calcium channel blockers, vasodilators, tricyclic antidepressants, digoxin, antiarrhythmic agents, and ß mimetic agents were not prmitted during the study.

Results

4 weeks of bisoprolol 10 mg/d reduced the mean number of transient ischemic episodes from 8.1±0.6 to 3.2±0.4 episodes/48 h (mean change -4.9, 95% CI -5.8 to -4.0). Nifedipine 20 mg X2/d reduced the number of ischemic episodes from 8.3±0.5 to 5.9±0.4 episodes/48 h (mean change -2.5, 95% CI -4.3 to -1.5). The effect of bisoprolol was almost twice that of nifedipine (bisoprolol vs nifedipine p=0.0001). Total duration of ischemic episodes were reduced from 99.3±10.1 to 31.9±5.5 min/48 h by bisoprolol (mean change -67.4, 95% CI -84.0 to -50.7), and from 101.0±9.1 to 72.6±8.1 min/48 h by nifedipine (mean change -28.4, 95% CI -45.9 to -10.9)(bisoprolol vs nifedipine p=0.0001). Doubling the dose of the medications resulted in only small additional effects that were significant only for bisoprolol. Bisoprolol reduced the heart rate at onset of ischemia by 13.7±1.4 bpm (p<0.001). Heart rate was not changed by nifedipine. 73.7% of the bisoprolol 10 mg/d vs 42.4% of the nifedipine 20 mg X2/d showed ≥50% reduction in the number of ischemic episodes (p<0.0001). The corresponding rates for the higher dose were 80.5% vs 49.2% (p<0.0001). Only bisoprolol showed a marked circadian effect by reducing the morning peak of ischemia.

Conclusions

Both agents reduced the number and duration of ischemic episodes in patients with stable angina. Bisoprolol was more effective than nifedipine.

IMAGE

International Multicenter Angina Exercise Study

Title	Combination therapy with metoprolol and nifedipine versus monotherapy in patients with stable angina pectoris. Results of the International Multicenter Angina Exercise (IMAGE) Study.
Authors	Savonitto S, Ardissino D, Egstrup K, et al.
Reference	J Am Coll Cardiol 1996;27:311-316
Disease	Angina pectoris
Purpose	To compare the efficacy of combination therapy with metoprolol and nifedipine versus either drug alone in patients with stable angina pectoris.
Design	Randomized, double blind, placebo controlled (second stage), multicenter.
Patients	280 patients, age ≤75 years, with stable angina for ≥6 months and a positive exercise test. Patients with myocardial infarction within 6 months, heart failure, inability to perform ≥3 min exercise test, or those with severe angina that preclude temporary cessation of medications, were excluded.
Follow-up	Exercise test at baseline, after the 6 weeks of monotherapy and after 10 weeks.
Treatment regimen	After 2-week placebo run-in period, patients were randomized to metoprolol 200 mg/d or nifedipine retard 20 mg X2/d for 6 weeks. Then, patients were randomized to addition of the second drug or placebo for 4 more weeks.

IMAGE

International Multicenter Angina Exercise Study

(continued)

Results

249 patients completed the study. By the end of 6 weeks the nifedipine treated group increased the mean duration of exercise time until 1 mm ST depression by 43 s compared with baseline (95% CI 16-69 s, $p<0.01$), and the metoprolol group by 70 s (95% CI 47-92 s, $p<0.01$). The improvement was greater with metoprolol ($p<0.05$). At week 10, the exercise time did not increase further in the patients who received placebo in addition to the metoprolol or nifedipine. However, addition of nifedipine to metoprolol resulted in further increase of the time (108 s more than in the baseline test (95% CI 71-145 s), and addition of metoprolol to nifedipine in 107 s (95% CI 64-151 s) more than in the baseline test ($p<0.05$ vs placebo). Analysis of the results in individual patients revealed that the additive effect was seen mainly in those who respond poorly to monotherapy.

Conclusions

Both drugs were effective as monotherapy in prolongation the exercise time (metoprolol more than nifedipine). The prolongation of exercise time, observed in the combination therapy, is not the result of an additive effect, but probably due to the effect of the second class of drug in patients not responding to the first one.

TREND

Trial on Reversing ENdothelial Dysfunction

Title	Angiotensin-converting enzyme inhibition with quinapril improves endothelial vasomotor dysfunction in patients with coronary artery disease. The TREND (trial on reversing endothelial dusfunction) study.
Authors	Mancini GBJ, Henry GC, Macaya C, et al.
Reference	Circulation 1996;94:258-265.
Disease	Coronary artery disease.
Purpose	To evaluate whether quinapril, an ACE inhibitor, improves endothelial dysfunction in normotensive patients with coronary artery disease and no heart failure, cardiomyopathy, or major lipid abnormalities.
Design	Randomized, double blind, placebo-controlled, multicenter.
Patients	129 patients, ≤75 years old, with documented coronary artery disease: single or double vessel disease (>50% diameter stenosis) that required a nonsurgical revascularization, and one adjacent coronary artery with <40% stenosis that had never been revascularized. This artery had to show endothelial dysfunction defined as either constriction or no response to acetylcholine. Patients with LDL cholesterol >165 mg/dL, hypertension (>160 mmHg systolic or >90 mmHg diastolic blood pressure), previous CABG, history of coronary spasm, coronary revascularization within 3 months, myocardial infarction within 7d, left ventricular ejection fraction <0.40, type I diabetes mellitus, valvular heart disease, hepatic or renal dysfunction, 2nd or 3rd degree AV block, or lipid lowering therapy within 6 months were excluded.
Follow-up	Cardiac catheterization with assessment of the response to intracoronary injection of acetylcholine 10^{-6} and 10^{-4} mol/L over 2 min before revascularization and after 6 months of therapy.

TREND

Trial on Reversing ENdothelial Dysfunction
(continued)

Treatment regimen	Quinapril 40 mg/d or placebo for 6 months.
Additional therapy	All vasoactive medications, except for ß-blockers and sublingual nitrates, were discontinued 12 h before angiography.
Results	105 patients underwent repeated angiography at 6 months. At baseline, before initiation of study medications, the constrictive response to acetylcholine was comparable between the placebo and quinapril groups (4.4% vs 6.1% after infusion of 10^{-6} mol/L, and 9.4% vs 14.3% after infusion of 10^{-4} mol/L (p=0.125), respectively). After 6 months of therapy there was no change in the response to acetylcholine in the placebo group (4.5% and 10.5% after acetylcholine 10^{-6} mol/L and 10^{-4} mol/L, respectively), whereas the quinapril-treated patients showed less constrictor response (1.6% and 2.3%, respectively) compared with the baseline study (p<0.014). Responses, expressed as net change from baseline, improved by 4.5±3.0% and 12.1±3.0% at each acetylcholine dose in the quinapril group, whereas the placebo group responses did not change (-0.1±2.8% and -0.8±2.9%, respectively, p<0.002). The analyses of the response to a nitroglycerin bolus (100-700 µg) revealed no difference between the groups at baseline (p=0.349) and after 6 months (p=0.336).
Conclusions	Angiotensin converting enzyme inhibition with quinapril improved endothelial function in normotensive patients without severe hyperlipidemia or heart failure.

4. Interventional Cardiology

a. PTCA or CABG Versus Medical Therapy

CASS

Coronary Artery Surgery Study

Title	a. Coronary artery surgery study (CASS): a randomized trial of coronary artery bypass surgery. Survival data. b. Myocardial infarction and mortality in the coronary artery surgery study (CASS) randomized trial. c. Ten-years follow-up of survival and myocardial infarction in the randomized coronary artery surgery study. d. Ten-year follow-up of quality of life in patients randomized to receive medical therapy or coronary artery bypass graft surgery. The coronary artery surgery study (CASS).
Authors	a.+b. CASS Principal Investigators and Their Associates. c. Alderman EL, Bourassa MG, Cohen LS, et al. d. Rogers WJ, Coggin CJ, Gersh BJ, et al.
Reference	a. Circulation 1983;68:939-950. b. N Engl J Med 1984;310:750-758. c. Circulation 1990;82:1629-1646. d. Circulation 1990;82:1647-1658.
Disease	Coronary artery disease, angina pectoris.
Purpose	To compare the effects of coronary artery bypass grafting surgery and medical therapy on mortality and morbidity in patients with mild angina or aymptomatic patients after myocardial infarction with coronary artery disease.
Design	Randomized, open label, multicenter.
Patients	780 patients, ≤65 years of age, with angina pectoris Canadian Cardiovascular Society Class I or II, or myocardial infarction >3 weeks before randomization. Patients with prior coronary bypass surgery, unstable angina, heart failure (NYHA class III or IV) were excluded.
Follow-up	10 years.

CASS

Coronary Artery Surgery Study

(continued)

Treatment regimen	Coronary artery bypass surgery or medical therapy.
Additional therapy	Common medical care including medications.
Results	The average annual mortality rate was 1.1% in the surgical group vs 1.6% in the medical group (p=NS). Annual mortality rates in patients with single-, double-, and three-vessel disease were 0.7% vs 1.4%, 1.0% vs 1.2%, and 1.5% vs 2.1%, in the surgical and medical groups respectively. The differences were not significant. The annual mortality rate for patients with ejection fraction <0.50 was 1.7% vs 3.3% in the surgical and medical groups. In these patients the probability of survival after 5 years was 83±4% in the medical vs 93±3% in the surgical groups (p=0.11). The annual rate of bypass surgery in the medical group was 4.7%. 6% had surgery within 6 months and 40% within 10 years. Nonfatal Q wave myocardial infarction occurred in 14% vs 11% in the surgical and medical group after 5 years (p=NS). The 5 year probability of remaining alive and free from infarction was 83% vs 82% (p=NS). There was no significant difference in survival or myocardial infarction curves between subgroups of patients assigned to medical vs surgical therapy. At 10 years 82% of the surgical vs 79% of the medical groups were alive (p=NS), and 66% vs 69%, respectively were free of death and myocardial infarction (p=NS). However, 79% vs 61% of the surgical and medical patients with initial ejection fraction <0.50 were alive after 10 years (p=0.01), while more patients with ejection fraction ≥0.50 on the medical therapy were free of death and infarction after 10 years (75% vs 68%, p=0.04). 66% vs 30%, 63% vs 38%, and 47% vs 42% of the surgical and medical groups were free from angina after 1, 5, and 10 years. By 5 years indexes of quality of life appeared superior in the surgery group. However, after 10 years the differences were less apparent.
Conclusions	Coronary bypass surgery did not prolong life or prevent myocardial infarction as compared with medical therapy in patients with mild angina or patients who are asymptomatic after myocardial infarction. However, long term survival was improved by surgical therapy in patients with initial ejection fraction <0.50.

ACME

Angioplasty Compared to Medicine

Title	A comparison of angioplasty with medical therapy in the treatment of single-vessel coronary artery disease.
Authors	Parisi AF, Folland ED, Hartigan P, et al.
Reference	N Engl J Med 1992;326:10-16.
Disease	Coronary artery disease, stable angina pectoris.
Purpose	To compare the results after 6 months of angioplasty versus medical therapy in patients with stable angina pectoris and single-vessel coronary artery disease.
Design	Randomized, multicenter.
Patients	212 patients with stable angina pectoris , positive exercise test, or myocardial infarction within the past 3 months, and 70-99% stenosis of the proximal 2/3 of a coronary artery.
Follow-up	Clinical evaluation every month. Exercise test and angiography after 6 months.
Treatment regimen	1. Medical therapy: a stepped-care approach including nitrates, ß-blockers, and calcium blockers. 2. Coronary angioplasty + calcium blocker for 1 month, and nitroglycerin during and for 12 h after the angioplasty.
Additional therapy	Oral aspirin 325 mg/d.

ACME

Angioplasty Compared to Medicine

(continued)

Results

Angioplasty was successful in 80 of the 100 patients who actually underwent the procedure. 2 patients in the angioplasty group required emergency coronary artery bypass surgery. After 6 months, 16 of the angioplasty group had repeated angioplasty. Of the 107 patients assigned to medical therapy, 11 underwent angioplasty. Myocardial infarction occurred in 5 and 3 of the patients assigned to angioplasty and medical therapy. After 6 months, 64% and 46% of the angioplasty and medical groups were free of angina ($p<0.01$). The angioplasty group were able to increase their total duration of exercise by 2.1 min, while the medical group by only 0.5 min ($p<0.0001$). The maximal heart rate-blood pressure product decreased by 2800 units in the medical group, while it increased by 1800 units in the angioplasty group ($p<0.0001$). The overall psychological-well-being score improved by 8.6 and 2.4 in the angioplasty and medical therapy groups ($p=0.03$).

Conclusions

Angioplasty offers earlier and better relief of angina than medical therapy and is associated with better performance on the exercise test in patients with single vessel disease. However, the initial costs and the complication rates are higher with angioplasty.

4. Interventional Cardiology
b. PTCA Versus CABG

RITA

Randomized Intervention Treatment of Angina (RITA) Trial

Title	a. The randomized intervention treatment of angina (RITA) trial protocol: a long-term study of coronary angioplasty and coronary artery bypass surgery in patients with angina. b. Coronary angioplasty versus coronary artery bypass surgery: the Randomized Intervention Treatment of Angina (RITA) trial. c. Health service costs of coronary angioplasty and coronary artery bypass surgery: the Randomized intervention Treatment of Angina (RITA) trial.
Authors	a. Henderson RA, for the RITA Trial. b. RITA Trial Participants. c. Sculpher MJ, Henderson RA, Buxton MJ, et al.
Reference	a. Br Heart J 1989;62:411-414. b. Lancet 1993;341:573-580. c. Lancet 1994;344:927-930.
Disease	Coronary artery disease.
Purpose	To compare the long term effects of percutaneous transluminal coronary angioplasty (PTCA) versus coronary artery bypass surgery (CABG) in patients with 1-, 2-, and 3-vessel disease.
Design	Randomized, multicenter.
Patients	1011 patients with coronary artery disease with a need for revascularization. Patients with left main coronary artery disease, previous PTCA or CABG, or significant valvular disease were excluded.
Follow-up	> 6 months, median 2.5 years.
Treatment regimen	CABG vs PTCA.

Randomized Intervention Treatment of Angina (RITA) Trial

(continued)

Results

Angioplasty was successful in 87% of the lesions. Emergency CABG was required in 4.5% of the PTCA group. Additional 1.4% underwent CABG before hospital discharge due to unsuccessful PTCA. Among the CABG patients 0.6% had pulmonary embolism and 4.9% wound-related complications. Median hospital stay was 12 and 4 days for CABG and PTCA, respectively. Mortality was 3.6% in the CABG and 3.1% in the PTCA group. Definite myocardial infarction occurred in 4.0% vs 6.5% of the CABG and PTCA patients. However, there was no difference in the rate of the primary end point (myocardial infarction or mortality) between the groups (RR CABG vs PTCA 0.88, 95% CI 0.59-1.29, p=0.47). Within 2 years an estimated 38% of the PTCA vs 11% of the CABG patients had experienced either further CABG, PTCA, myocardial infarction, or death (p<0.001). The prevalence of angina during follow-up was 32% in the PTCA vs 11% in the CABG group after 6 months (RR 0.35, 95% CI 0.26-0.47, p<0.001) and 31% vs 22% after 2 years (p=0.007).

Conclusions

While there was no difference in mortality, CABG was associated with less recurrent angina and need for revascularization.

ERACI

Argentine Randomized Trial of Percutaneous Transluminal Coronary Angioplasty versus Coronary Artery Bypass Surgery in Multivessel Disease.

Title	Argentine randomized trial of percutaneous transluminal coronary angioplasty versus coronary artery bypass surgery in multivessel disease (ERACI): in-hospital results and 1-year follow-up.
Authors	Rodriguez A, Boullon F, Perez-Baliño N, et al.
Reference	J Am Coll Cardiol 1993;22:1060-1067.
Disease	Coronary artery disease.
Purpose	To compare outcome following coronary artery bypass surgery (CABG) vs percutaneous transluminal coronary angioplasty (PTCA) in patients with multivessel coronary artery disease.
Design	Randomized, one center.
Patients	127 patients, age 33-76 years, with stable angina and multivessel disease which was suitable to either PTCA or CABG.
Follow-up	1 year clinical follow-up.
Treatment regimen	CABG vs PTCA.

ERACI

Argentine Randomized Trial of Percutaneous Transluminal Coronary Angioplasty versus Coronary Artery Bypass Surgery in Multivessel Disease.

(continued)

Results

The overall primary success rate of angioplasty was 91.7% per lesion. There was no significant difference in in-hospital mortality (4.6% vs 1.5%), myocardial infarction (6.2% vs 6.3%), stroke (3.1% vs 1.5%), or need for repeated emergency procedure (1.5% vs 1.5%) between the CABG and the PTCA groups. Complete revascularization was achieved in 88% vs 51% of the CABG and PTCA groups ($p<0.001$). Mortality after 1 year was 3.2% in the PTCA vs 0% in the CABG patients (p=NS). New Q wave infarction occurred in 3.2% of the PTCA and 1.8% of the CABG (p=NS). 32% of the PTCA group needed revascularization vs 3.2% of the CABG patients ($p<0.001$). However, freedom from angina (including patients with repeated procedure) after 1 year was similar.

Conclusions

No significant differences were found in major in-hospital complications and 1 year outcome between the groups. However, after 1 year more patients treated with PTCA needed repeated revascularization.

GABI

The German Angioplasty Bypass Surgery Investigation

Title	A randomized study of coronary angioplasty compared with bypass surgery in patients with symptomatic multivessel coronary disease.
Authors	Hamm CW, Reimers J, Ischinger T, et al.
Reference	N Engl J Med 1994;331:1037-1043.
Disease	Coronary artery disease.
Purpose	To compare the outcomes of coronary revascularization with coronary artery bypass grafting (CABG) and percutaneous transluminal coronary angioplasty (PTCA) in patients with multivessel disease.
Design	Randomized, multicenter.
Patients	337 patients, <75 years old, with symptomatic multivessel disease (Canadian Cardiovascular Society class ≥II, and ≥70% stenosis), and a need for revascularization of ≥2 major coronary arteries. Patients with 100% occlusion or >30% stenosis of the left main coronary artery were excluded. Patients who underwent prior CABG or PTCA and patients with myocardial infarction within 4 weeks were excluded.
Follow-up	1 year.
Treatment regimen	CABG vs PTCA.

GABI

The German Angioplasty Bypass Surgery Investigation

(continued)

Results

Among the CABG patients an average of 2.2±0.6 vessels were grafted, and among the PTCA patients 1.9±0.5 vessels were dilated. Complete revascularization was achieved in 86% of the PTCA patients. Hospitalization was longer after CABG (median days 19 vs 5), and Q wave infarction related to the procedure was more common (8.1% vs 2.3%, p=0.022). However, there was no significant difference in mortality (2.5% vs 1.1%, p=0.43). At discharge 93% vs 82% of the CABG and PTCA patients were angina-free (p=0.005). During the following year 6% of the CABG patients vs 44% of the PTCA patients underwent repeated interventions (p<0.001). The cumulative risk of death or myocardial infarction was 13.6% in the CABG and 6.0% in the PTCA patients (p=0.017). One year after the procedure 74% vs 71%, respectively were angina-free (p=NS). Exercise capacity was similar. However, 22% of the CABG vs only 12% of the PTCA patients did not require antianginal medication (p=0.041). 219 patients underwent coronary angiography after 6 months. The clinical course of these patients did not differ from that of those who refused to undergo repeated catheterization. 13% of the vein grafts were occluded and 7% of the internal thoracic artery anastomoses did not function, whereas 16% of the vessels dilated by angioplasty were ≥70% stenotic.

Conclusions

In selected patients with multivessel disease PTCA and CABG resulted in similar improvement after 1 year. However, the PTCA treated patients needed more additional interventions and antianginal medication, whereas CABG was more associated with procedure related myocardial infarction.

EAST

The Emory Angioplasty Versus Surgery Trial

Title	a. A randomized trial comparing coronary angioplasty with coronary bypass surgery. b. A comparison of the costs of and quality of life after coronary angioplasty or coronary surgery for multivessel coronary artery disease: results from the Emory Angioplasty versus Surgery Trial (EAST).
Authors	a. King SB III, Lembo NJ, Weintraub WS, et al. b. Weintraub WS, Mauldin PD, Becker E, et al.
Reference	a. N Engl J Med 1994;331:1044-1050. b. Circulation 1995;92:2831-2840.
Disease	Coronary artery disease.
Purpose	To compare the outcome following coronary artery bypass surgery (CABG) vs percutaneous transluminal coronary angioplasty (PTCA) in patients with multivessel coronary artery disease.
Design	Randomized, single center.
Patients	392 patients of any age with 2- to 3-vessel disease and had not previously undergone PTCA or CABG. Patients with old 100% occlusion of vessels serving viable myocardium, ≥2 total occlusions, >30% left main artery stenosis, ejection fraction ≤25%, or myocardial infarction <5 d, were excluded.
Follow-up	3 year clinical follow-up. Repeated angiography and thallium scan after 1 and 3 years.
Treatment regimen	PTCA vs CABG.

EAST

The Emory Angioplasty Versus Surgery Trial

(continued)

Results

In hospital mortality was 1.0% in each group. Q wave infarction occurred in 10.3% of the CABG and 3.0% of the PTCA patients (p=0.004). Stroke occurred in 1.5% vs 0.5%, respectively (p=0.37). 0% and 10.1% of the patients, respectively underwent emergency CABG during hospitalization. 3 year mortality was 6.2% in the CABG and 7.1% in the PTCA groups (p=0.72). Q wave infarction within 3 years occurred in 19.6% vs 14.6%, respectively (p=0.21). Large ischemic defect on thallium scan were found in 5.7% vs 9.6%, respectively (p=0.17). There was no difference in the occurrence of the composite end point (death, Q wave infarction, or a large ischemic defect on thallium scan)(27.3% vs 28.8%, p=0.81). After 3 years 1% of the CABG vs 22% of the PTCA group underwent CABG (p<0.001), while PTCA was performed in 13% vs 41%, respectively (p<0.001). Initially, 99.1% vs 75.1% of the index segments per patients were revascularized in the CABG and PTCA, respectively. 1 year later, 88.1% vs 58.8% of the index segment per patients were revascularized (p<0.001). However, by 3 years the differences were narrowed (86.7% vs 69.9%, respectively, p<0.001). There was no difference in ejection fraction between the groups. However, angina was present in 12% and 20% of the patients after 3 years, respectively.

Conclusions

PTCA and CABG did not differ significantly with respect to the occurrence of the composite end points. However, PTCA was associated with more repeated procedures and residual angina.

CABRI

Coronary Angioplasty Versus Bypass Revascularization Investigation

Title	First-year results of CABRI (Coronary Angioplasty versus Bypass Revascularization Investigation).
Authors	CABRI Trial Participants.
Reference	Lancet 1995;346:1179-1184.
Disease	Coronary artery disease.
Purpose	To compare the effects of percutaneous transluminal coronary angioplasty (PTCA) vs coronary artery bypass surgery (CABG) in patients with multivessel disease.
Design	Randomized, multicenter.
Patients	1054 patients, <76 years old, with >1 vessel disease with left ventricular ejection fraction >0.35. Patients with left main or severe triple vessel disease, overt cardiac failure, myocardial infarction within 10 days, a previous coronary revascularization or a recent cerebrovascular event were excluded. At least one lesion had to be suitable for PTCA.
Follow-up	1 year.
Treatment regimen	CABG or PTCA (stents and atherectomy were permitted).
Additional therapy	Aspirin. The use of fish oil and lipid-lowering agents were allowed.

CABRI

Coronary Angioplasty Versus Bypass Revascularization Investigation

(continued)

Results

After 1 year 2.7% of the CABG and 3.9% of the PTCA allocated patients had died (RR 1.42, 95% CI 0.73-2.76, $p=0.3$). Kaplan-Meier survival curves did not demonstrate a difference in survival at 28 months. The PTCA allocated group required more repeated interventions. 20.8% vs 2.7% needed angioplasty, while 15.7% vs 0.8% needed CABG. 66.4% of the PTCA vs 93.5% of the CABG group had only a single procedure in the first year. The rate of reintervention was 5 times higher in the PTCA group (RR 5.23, 95% CI 3.90-7.03, $p<0.001$). The PTCA group needed more antianginal medications (RR 1.30, 95% CI 1.18-1.43, $p<0.001$). After 1 year 67 % of the PTCA vs 75% of the CABG were angina-free .The presence of angina at 1 year was greater in the PTCA than in the CABG group (RR 1.54, 95% CI 1.09-2.16, $p=0.012$).

Conclusions

CABG as the initial revascularization strategy for multivessel disease was associated with decreased need for repeated procedure. However, one-year survival was similar.

BARI

The Bypass Angioplasty Revascularization Investigation

Title	a. Comparison of coronary bypass surgery with angioplasty in patients with multivessel disease. b. Five-year clinical and functional outcome comparing bypass surgery and angioplasty in patients with multivessel coronary disease. A multicenter randomized trial.
Authors	The Bypass Angioplasty Revascularization Investigation (BARI) Investigators.
Reference	a. N Engl J Med 1996;335:217-225. b. JAMA 1997;277:715-721.
Disease	Coronary artery disease.
Purpose	To compare the long term effects of percutaneous transluminal coronary balloon angioplasty (PTCA) and coronary artery bypass grafting surgery (CABG) in patients with multivessel coronary artery disease.
Design	Randomized, multicenter.
Patients	1829 patients with angiographically documented multivessel coronary artery disease, with clinically severe angina or evidence of ischemia requiring revascularization, and were suitable for both PTCA and CABG.
Follow-up	Mean follow-up 5.4 years (range 3.8 to 6.8 years).
Treatment regimen	PTCA vs CABG. New interventional devices, such as stents and atherectomy devices were not used during the initial revascularization procedure.
Results	Of the 915 patients randomized to PTCA, 904 (99%) actually underwent the procedure, 9 underwent CABG, and 2 received medical therapy alone. Of the 914 patients randomized to CABG, 892 (98%) underwent the procedure,

15 underwent PTCA as the initial procedure, and 7 were treated medically. Among the 892 patients who underwent CABG as assigned, an average of 3.1 coronary arteries were bypassed with a mean of 2.8 grafts. In 91% of patients all intended vessels were revascularized. At least one internal-thoracic-artery was used in 82% of patients. Among the 904 patients who underwent PTCA as assigned, angioplasty was attempted on an average of 2.4 lesions. Multilesion angioplasty was attempted in 78% of patients, and multivessel angioplasty in 70% of patients. Immediate angiographic success was achieved in 78% of the attempted angioplasties. Rates of in-hospital mortality were comparable between the CABG and PTCA groups (1.3% vs 1.1% in the CABG and PTCA group, respectively; p=NS). Q wave myocardial infarction during hospitalization occurred in 4.6% vs 2.1%, respectively ($p<0.01$). There was no statistically significant difference between the groups in the occurrence of stroke, congestive heart failure, cardiogenic shock, and nonfatal cardiac arrest. However, more of the CABG patients experienced respiratory failure (2.2% vs 1.0%, $p<0.05$), wound dehiscence or infection (4.1% vs 0.4%, $p<0.001$), and reoperation for bleeding (3.1% vs 0.4%, $p<0.001$). Emergency CABG (6.3% vs 0.1%; $p<0.001$) and PTCA (2.1% vs 0; $p<0.001$) following the initial procedure were performed more often in the PTCA group. Nonemergency CABG was also performed more often in the PTCA patients (3.9% vs 0; $p<0.001$). The median hospital stay was longer after CABG (7 days) than after PTCA (3 days). The cumulative survival rates at five years were 89.3% and 86.3% for the CABG and PTCA groups, respectively (2.9% difference, 95% CI -0.2% to 6.0%; p=0.19). The cumulative rates of Q wave myocardial infarction at five years were 11.7% and 10.9%, respectively (p=0.45). At five years 80.4% and 78.7% of the CABG and PTCA patients were alive and free of Q wave myocardial infarction (1.6% difference, 95% confidence interval -2.2% to 5.4%, p=0.84). During the 5-year follow-up, 8% of the CABG patients underwent repeated revascularization procedures (1% underwent repeated CABG and 7% PTCA), while 54% of the PTCA group underwent at least one additional procedure (31% underwent CABG and 34% repeated PTCA, 11% underwent both CABG and PTCA). Multiple additional revascularization procedures were required for 19% of the PTCA patients versus 3% of the CABG patients. Patients undergoing PTCA had more frequent hospitalizations than the CABG patients (an aver-

age of 2.5 per patient versus 1.9, p<0.001). At 4 to 14 weeks 95% of the CABG vs 73% of the PTCA patients reported no angina (p<0.001). At the 5-year visit 86% of the CABG vs 78% of the PTCA patients were angina-free (p=0.003). At 4 to 14 weeks visit, 20% of the CABG vs 31% of the PTCA group had abnormal exercise-induced ST segment changes (p<0.001), however, at 5 years there was no difference (28% vs 31%). At five years there was no difference in the proportion of patients experiencing exercise induced angina. During follow-up, patients in the PTCA were more likely to receive anti-ischemic medications than the CABG group (89% vs 44% at 4-14 weeks (p<0.001), 76% vs 57% by the fifth year (p<0.001). At follow-up of 1 year and later, quality of life, return to work, modification of smoking and exercise behaviors, and cholesterol levels were similar for the two groups. Subgroup analysis did not reveal a difference in survival between CABG and PTCA in patients with unstable angina or non-Q wave infarction, stable angina, severe ischemia, normal or reduced left ventricular function, double or triple vessel disease, and presence of type C coronary lesions (complicated lesions). However, a significant survival benefit was observed in patients with treated diabetes mellitus assigned to CABG. The 5-year survival in diabetic patients was 80.6% in the CABG compared to 65.5% in the PTCA group (15.1% difference, 99.5% confidence interval 1.4% to 28.9%, p=0.003).

Conclusions

The 5-year survival of patients assigned to initial strategy of PTCA was comparable to that of patients assigned to CABG. However, subsequent repeated revascularization was required more often in the PTCA group. In patients with diabetes mellitus, 5-year survival was significantly worse with PTCA than with CABG.

4. Interventional Cardiology
c. PTCA Versus Other Percutaneous Devices

CAVEAT-1

Coronary Angioplasty Versus Excisional Atherectomy Trial

Title	a. A comparison of directional atherectomy with coronary angioplasty in patients with coronary artery disease. b. One-year follow-up in the coronary angioplasty versus excisional atherectomy trial (CAVEAT I).
Authors	a. Topol EJ, Leya F, Pinkerton CA, et al. b.Elliott JM, Berdan LG, Holmes DR, et al.
Reference	a. N Engl J Med 1993;329:221-227. b. Circulation 1995;91:2158-2166.
Disease	Coronary artery disease; angina pectoris.
Purpose	To compare outcome of percutaneous transluminal coronary angioplasty (PTCA) with that of directional coronary atherectomy (DCA).
Design	Randomized, controlled trial.
Patients	1012 patients (median age 59 years, 73% men) with symptomatic coronary artery disease. Only patients with angiography-proven native coronary artery lesions ≥60% stenosis, and <12 mm length, with no prior intracoronary interventions were included. Patients who had acute myocardial infarction within 5 days of procedure were excluded. 512 and 500 patients were assigned to DCA and PTCA, respectively.
Follow-up	1 year.
Treatment regimen	Percutaneous transluminal coronary angioplasty (PTCA) or directional coronary atherectomy (DCA).

CAVEAT-1

Coronary Angioplasty Versus Excisional Atherectomy Trial

(continued)

Additional therapy

All patients received before procedure ≥160 mg aspirin, ≥1 dose of calcium channel blocker, and heparin as a bolus of 10000 U with additional boluses to maintain clotting time >350 sec during the procedure.

Results

Reduction of stenosis to ≤50% was more successful with DCA (89%) than PTCA (80%), $p<0.001$. The success rates (≤50% residual stenosis and no major complications) were higher in the DCA group (82%) than the PTCA group (76%, $p=0.016$). The immediate gain in luminal diameter was greater in the DCA (1.05 mm) than PTCA (0.86 mm, $p<0.001$) patients. However, early complications were more frequent in the DCA than PTCA patients (11% versus 5%, $p<0.001$). At six month 50% and 57% of the DCA and PTCA patients had restenosis, respectively ($p=0.06$). One-year mortality was 2.2% and 0.6% in the DCA and PTCA groups, respectively ($p=0.035$). Myocardial infarction within one year occurred in 8.9% of the DCA and 4.4% of the PTCA patients ($p=0.005$). By multivariate analysis, DCA was the only variable predictive of the combined end point of death or myocardial infarction. Rates of repeated interventions at the target site were similar.

Conclusions

DCA, as compared with PTCA, was associated with an increase rates of restenosis at 6 months, and one-year mortality and occurrence of myocardial infarction.

Directional Atherectomy vs Balloon Angioplasty for Lesions of the Left Anterior Descending Coronary Artery

Title	A comparison of directional atherectomy with balloon angioplasty for lesions of the left anterior descending coronary artery.
Authors	Adelman AG, Cohen EA, Kimball BP, et al.
Reference	N Engl J Med 1993;329:228-233.
Disease	Coronary artery disease, restenosis.
Purpose	To compare the rates of restenosis for directional atherectomy and balloon angioplasty in lesions of the proximal left anterior descending coronary artery.
Design	Randomized, open label, multicenter.
Patients	274 patients with de novo ≥60% stenosis of the proximal 1/3 of the left anterior descending coronary artery. Patients within 7 d of acute infarction or severe left ventricular dysfunction were excluded.
Follow-up	Clinical evaluation and repeated angiography at 4-7 months (median 5.9 months).
Treatment regimen	Directional atherectomy or balloon angioplasty.
Additional therapy	Aspirin, calcium channel blocker, and nitrates were started ≥12 h before procedure and continued for 24 h. Heparin was given during procedure. Antianginal medications were discontinued. The use of n-3 fatty acids was prohibited.

Results The procedural success rate was 94% in the atherectomy and 88% in the angioplasty patients (p=0.06). Major in-hospital complications occurred in 5% and 6%, respectively. Repeated angiography was performed in 257 patients. After 6 months, the restenosis rate was 46% and 43% (p=0.7). Despite a greater initial gain in minimal luminal diameter (1.45±0.47 vs 1.16±0.44 mm, p<0.001), there was a larger loss (0.79±0.61 vs 0.47±0.64 mm, p<0.001) in the atherectomy group, resulting in a similar minimal luminal diameter at follow-up (1.55±0.60 vs 1.61±0.68 mm, p=0.44). The clinical outcome was similar in the two groups.

Conclusions Despite better initial success rate and gain in minimal luminal diameter, atherectomy did not result in better clinical outcome or late angiographic results with lesions of the proximal third of the left anterior descending coronary artery.

Title	a. A comparison of balloon-expandable stent implantation with balloon angioplasty in patients with coronary artery disease. b. Continued benefit of coronary stenting versus balloon angioplasty: one-year clinical follow-up of Benestent Trial.
Authors	a. Serruys PW, de Jaegere P, Kiemenij F, et al. b. Macay a C, Serruys PW, Ruygrok P, et al.
Reference	a. N Engl J Med 1994;331:489-495. b. J Am Coll Cardiol 1996;27:255-261.
Disease	Coronary artery disease, restenosis.
Purpose	To compare elective balloon angioplasty with Palmaz-Schatz stent implantation in patients with stable angina and de novo coronary artery lesions.
Design	Randomized, multicenter.
Patients	516 patients, age 30-75 years, with stable angina and a single new lesion of the native coronary circulation <15 mm, located in vessels >3 mm and supplying normally functioning myocardium.
Follow-up	12 months (0.3-34 months). Exercise test and repeated angiography at 6 months.
Treatment regimen	Balloon angioplasty or Palmaz-Schatz stent implantation.
Additional therapy	Aspirin 250-500 mg/d and dipyridamole 75 mg X3/d, started ≥1 d before procedure and continued for >6 months. IV heparin 10,000 U bolus before procedure. calcium channel blockers until discharge. Patients undergoing stent implantation received dextran infusion (1,000 ml over 6-8 h), heparin infusion (started after sheath removal and continued for ≥36 h), and warfarin for 3 months (target INR 2.5-3.5).

Results

The procedural success rate was 92.7% in the stent group and 91.1% in the angioplasty group, whereas the angiographic success was 96.9% vs 98.1%, respectively. There was no differences in the incidence of death, stroke, myocardial infarction, or the need for repeated procedures during the index hospitalization between the groups. There was no difference in the composite end point of all in-hospital clinical events (6.2% in the angioplasty vs 6.9% in the stent group (RR 1.12, 95% CI 0.58-2.14)). Subacute vessel closure occurred in 2.7% of the angioplasty and 3.5% of the stent group (p=NS). The incidence of bleeding and vascular complications was higher in the stent group 13.5% vs 3.1%, RR 4.34, 95% CI 2.05-9.18, p<0.001). Mean hospitalization was 8.5±6.8 days in the stent vs 3.1±3.3 days in the angioplasty group (p=0.001). After 7 months primary events occurred in 29.6% vs 20.1% of the angioplasty and stent groups (RR 0.68, 95% CI 0.50-0.92, p=0.02). The major difference was the need for repeated angioplasty in the angioplasty group (20.6% vs 10.0%, RR 0.49, 95% CI 0.31-0.75, p=0.001).The minimal luminal diameter after the procedure was 2.48±0.39 vs 2.05±0.33 mm (p<0.001), and at follow-up it was 1.82± 0.64 vs 1.73±0.55 mm (p=0.09), in the stent and angioplasty groups. The incidence of >50% restenosis was 22% vs 32%, respectively (p=0.02). After 1 year a primary end point occurred in 32% of the angioplasty vs 23% of the stent group (RR 0.74, 95% CI 0.55-0.98, p=0.04). However, the only significant difference was the rate of repeated interventions.

Conclusions

Implantation of stent is associated with better initial gain in luminal stenosis, a larger minimal diameter after 7 months and a significant reduction of the need for repeated interventions that was maintained to at least one year. However, stent implantation is associated with longer hospital stay and more bleeding and vascular complications.

STRESS

Stent Restenosis Study

Title	A randomized comparison of coronary-stent placement and balloon angioplasty in the treatment of coronary artery disease.
Authors	Fischman DL, Leon MB, Baim DS, et al.
Reference	N Engl J Med 1994;331:496-501.
Disease	Coronary artery disease, restenosis.
Purpose	To compare the results of Palmaz-Schatz stent placement and conventional balloon angioplasty on restenosis and clinical outcome.
Design	Randomized, open label, multicenter.
Patients	407 patients with new ≥70% stenotic lesions, ≤15 mm in length, in ≥3.0 mm of a native coronary artery. Patients with myocardial infarction within 7 days, ejection fraction <40%, diffuse coronary or left main artery disease, or angiographic evidence of thrombus were excluded.
Follow-up	Clinical follow-up for 6 months. Repeated angiography at 6 months.
Treatment regimen	Palmaz-Schatz stent placement or balloon angioplasty.

Additional therapy For the stent arm: Aspirin 325 mg/d and dipyridamole 75 mg X3/d and calcium channel blocker. IV low-molecular weight dextran started 2 h before procedure at a dose of 100 ml/h for 2 h, and during and after procedure 50 ml/h. IV heparin 10,000-15,000 U before procedure, and IV infusion 4-6 h after removal of the sheath. Warfarin sodium started on the day of procedure. Dipyridamole and warfarin were administered for 1 month, and aspirin indefinitely. For the angioplasty arm: Aspirin 325 mg/d, without warfarin sodium or dipyridamole.

Results Clinical success was achieved in 96.1% and 89.6% of the stent and angioplasty groups ($p=0.011$). The stent group had a larger immediate gain in minimal diameter of the lumen (1.72±0.46 vs 1.23±0.48 mm, $p<0.001$), and a larger luminal diameter after the procedure (2.49±0.43 vs 1.99±0.47 mm, $p<0.001$). There was no statistical significant difference in the rate of any of the early clinical events (days 0-14) between the groups. At 6 months, the stent group had a larger luminal diameter (1.74±0.60 vs 1.56±0.65 mm, $p=0.007$), and a lower rate of ≥50% restenosis (31.6% vs 42.1%, $p=0.046$). 80.5% and 76.2% of the stent and angioplasty groups were event-free after 6 months ($p=0.16$). Revascularization of the original lesion was performed in 10.2% and 15.4% of the stent and angioplasty patients ($p=0.06$).

Conclusions In selected patients, placement of Palmaz-Schatz stent was associated with better immediate results, lower rate of 6 months restenosis, and less revascularization procedures.

CAVEAT-II

Coronary Angioplasty Versus Directional Atherectomy- II

Title	A multicenter, randomized trial of coronary angioplasty versus directional atherectomy for patients with saphenous vein bypass graft lesions.
Authors	Holmes DR, Topol EJ, Califf RM, et al.
Reference	Circulation 1995;91:1966-1974.
Disease	Coronary artery disease, saphenous vein grafts.
Purpose	To compare outcome after directional coronary atherectomy versus angioplasty in patients with de novo venous bypass graft stenosis.
Design	Randomized, open label, multicenter.
Patients	305 patients with de novo saphenous vein graft lesions, ≥60% and <100% stenosis, who required revascularization and were suitable for either angioplasty or atherectomy.
Follow-up	Clinical evaluation and repeated coronary angiography at 6 months.
Treatment regimen	Balloon angioplasty or directional atherectomy.
Additional therapy	Aspirin ≥160 mg and a calcium blocker <24 h before procedure. A bolus of 10,000 U heparin before procedure. Aspirin 325 mg/d and a calcium channel blocker for 1 month.

Results Initial angiographic success was 89.2% with atherectomy vs 79.0% with angioplasty (p=0.019), as was initial luminal gain (1.45 vs 1.12 mm, p<0.001). Distal embolization occurred in 13.4% and 5.1% of the patients, respectively (p=0.012), and non-Q wave infarction in 16.1% and 9.6%, respectively (p=0.09). The restenosis rates (>50% stenosis) were similar at 6 months (45.6% vs 50.5%, p=0.49). 13.2% of the atherectomy and 22.4% of the angioplasty patients required repeated interventions (p=0.41).

Conclusions Atherectomy of de novo vein graft lesion was associated with better initial angiographic success, but with increased distal embolization. There was no difference in restenosis rates, however, there was a trend towards less target-vessel revascularization procedures.

AMRO

Amsterdam-Rotterdam trial

Title	Randomised trial of excimer laser angioplasty versus balloon angioplasty for treatment of obstructive coronary artery disease
Authors	Appelman YEA, Piek JJ, Strikwerda S, et al.
Reference	Lancet 1996;347:79-84.
Disease	Coronary artery disease, restenosis.
Purpose	To compare the initial and 6-month clinical and angiographic outcome of excimer laser coronary angioplasty versus balloon angioplasty.
Design	Randomized, multicenter.
Patients	308 patients with stable angina pectoris, coronary lesions >10 mm, or total or functional occlusions (TIMI flow grade 0 or 1), either with single or multivessel disease) who were suitable for coronary angioplasty. Patients with unstable angina; myocardial infarction within 2 weeks; a life expectancy of <1 year; intended angioplasty of a venous graft; unprotected left main disease angulated, highly eccentric, ostial or bifurcation lesions; lesions with a thrombus or dissection; and total occlusions with low likelihood of passage with a guide wire were excluded.
Follow-up	Clinical follow up and repeated coronary angiography at 6 months.
Treatment regimen	Excimer laser angioplasty (wave-length 308 nm) or balloon angioplasty (PTCA)

AMRO

Amsterdam-Rotterdam trial

(continued)

Additional therapy

Nifedipine 20 mgX3/d during hospitalization. Aspirin 250-500 mg/d, started a day before the procedure and continued for 6 months. Intravenous heparin for ≥12 h after procedure.

Results

155 patients (162 lesions) were randomized to excimer laser, and 158 patients (162 lesions) to PTCA. In 5 patients, the randomized segment was not treated. Excimer laser could not be done in 25 patients. Of the remaining 133 lesions, 98% (130 lesions) were treated with additional PTCA. Of the 167 lesions (157 patients) assigned to PTCA, PTCA was not done in 24 patients due to inability to cross the lesion. The angiographic success rate was 80% after laser and 79% after PTCA. There were no deaths. Myocardial infarction occurred in 4.6% vs 5.7% of the excimer laser and PTCA groups, respectively (p=0.67). There was no difference in the rates of coronary artery bypass surgery (10.6% vs 10.8%, respectively; p=0.95), repeated angioplasty (21.2% in the laser vs 18.5% in the PTCA group; p=0.55), or in the occurrence of primary endpoint (death, myocardial infarction, or repeated revascularization; 33.1% vs 29.9%; p=0.55). The incidence of transient occlusions of the randomized segment was higher in the excimer laser (10 patients) than PTCA (1 patient) (relative risk 10.57; 95% CI 1.37 to 81.62; p=0.005). Arterial diameter stenosis was comparable between the groups before procedure, immediately after and at follow up. The restenosis (>50% diameter) rate was higher in the excimer laser group (51.6% vs 41.3%; difference 10.3%; 95% CI -2.0% to 22.6%; p=0.13). Minimal lumen diameter in the excimer laser and PTCA groups were 0.77±0.44 vs 0.77±0.47 mm before procedure, 1.69±0.41 vs 1.59±0.34 mm immediately after procedure (p=0.05), and 1.17±0.71 vs 1.25±0.68 mm at follow-up (p=0.34). Net gain in lumen minimal diameter (at follow-up minus before procedure) tended to be larger with PTCA (0.48±0.66 vs 0.40±0.69 mm; p=0.34). Late minimal lumen diameter loss (immediately after procedure minus at follow-up) was greater with excimer laser (0.52±0.70 vs 0.34±0.62 mm; 0.18 mm difference; 95% CI 0.15 to 0.35; p=0.04).

Conclusions

Excimer laser coronary angioplasty followed by PTCA was not better than conventional PTCA alone in the treatment of obstructive coronary lesions.

SICCO

Stenting In Chronic Coronary Occlusion

Title	Stenting in chronic coronary occlusion (SICCO): a randomized, controlled trial of adding stent implantation after successful angioplasty.
Authors	Sirnes PA, Golf S, Myreng Y, et al.
Reference	J Am Coll Cardiol 1996;28:1444-1451.
Disease	Coronary artery disease, restenosis.
Purpose	To investigate whether stent implantation improves long-term results after recanalization by angioplasty of chronic coronary artery occlusions.
Design	Randomized, multicenter.
Patients	117 patients, >18 years old, who underwent conventional balloon angioplasty (PTCA) of an occluded native coronary artery (TIMI flow grade 0 or I). Patients with occlusion of <2 weeks old, inability to tolerate anticoagulant therapy, reference artery diameter <2.5 mm, major dissection following angioplasty, elastic recoil >50% after angioplasty, lesions with complex anatomy, poor distal runoff, or angiographically visible thrombus were excluded.
Follow-up	Repeated coronary angiography after 6 months.
Treatment regimen	After conventional successful PTCA, patients were randomized to either a control group with no additional intervention, or to Palmaz-Schatz stent implantation.

Additional therapy

Aspirin 75 to 160 mg/d, started before angioplasty, heparin 10,000 to 15,000 IU before PTCA and then heparin infusion for 12 to 24 h in the control group and for 2 to 5 days in the stented group. The patients in the stent group received an infusion of dextran (1000 ml, 50 ml/h). The stented patients received dipyridamole 75 mgX3/d and warfarin (INR 3.5 to 4.0) for 3 months.

Results

There were no deaths throughout the follow-up period. Stent delivery was unsuccessful in one patient. One patient with stent implantation had a myocardial infarction. Stent implantation resulted in an increase in minimal luminal diameter from 2.21±0.50 to 2.78±0.49 mm ($p<0.001$). Vessel closure within 14 days occurred in 6.9% and 5.1% of the stent and control groups (p=NS). Inguinal hematoma was more common in the stent group (11 vs 0 patients; $p=0.04$). At follow-up, 57% vs 24% of the stent and control groups had no angina ($p<0.001$). There was no difference in late target revascularization during the 6 month follow-up (3 patients in each group), however, at 300 days after the procedure more patients in the control than stent group underwent repeated revascularization (42.4% vs 22.4%). Follow-up angiography was performed in 114 patients. ≥50% diameter stenosis developed in 32% vs 74% of the stent and control group, respectively (Odds ratio 0.165; 95% CI 0.07 to 0.37; $p<0.001$); reocclusion occurred in 12% vs 26%, respectively ($p=0.058$). Minimal luminal diameter at follow-up was larger in the stent group (1.92±0.95 vs 1.11±0.78 mm; $p<0.001$).

Conclusions

Stent implantation after successful balloon angioplasty of chronic coronary artery occlusions improved long-term angiographic results, and was associated with less recurrence of angina and less revascularization procedures.

4. Interventional Cardiology

d. Medical Therapy to Prevent Restenosis after Intracoronary Interventions or Occlusion After Coronary Artery Bypass Grafting

CARPORT

Coronary Artery Restenosis Prevention on Repeated Thromboxane-Antagonism Study

Title	Prevention of restenosis after percutaneous transluminal coronary angioplasty with thromboxane A2-receptor blockade. A randomized, double-blind, placebo-controlled trial.
Authors	Serruys PW, Rutsch W, Heyndrick GR, et al.
Reference	Circulation 1991;84:1568-1580.
Disease	Coronary artery disease, restenosis.
Purpose	To evaluate the efficacy of GR32191B, a thromboxane A2-receptor antagonist, to prevent restenosis following coronary angioplasty.
Design	Randomized, double-blind, placebo-controlled, multicenter.
Patients	697 patients, >21 years old, with coronary artery disease who were excluded for angioplasty for de novo lesions in native arteries. Patients with myocardial infarction within 2 weeks of procedure were excluded.
Follow-up	Clinical evaluation, exercise test, and repeated angiography at 6 months.
Treatment regimen	1. GR32191B 80 mg PO 1 h + saline infusion before procedure. 40 mg X2/d GR32191B thereafter. 2. Placebo PO + 250 mg aspirin IV before procedure. Placebo X2/d thereafter. Aspirin and NSAID were prohibited during the follow-up.
Additional therapy	Heparin IV 10,000 U bolus, 10 mg nifedipine every 2 h for 12 h, and then 20 mg of slow released nifedipine X3/d for 2 days.

CARPORT

Coronary Artery Restenosis Prevention on Repeated Thromboxane-Antagonism Study

(continued)

Results

522 compliant patients underwent repeated angiography. The mean minimal luminal diameter loss was 0.31±0.54 vs 0.31±0.55 mm in the control and treated group. A loss of ≥0.72 mm was found in 19% and 21% of the patients, respectively. 6 months after procedure 72% and 75% of the patients, respectively were symptom free. There was no difference in the rates of clinical events during the 6 months between the groups. There was no difference in exercise performance between the groups.

Conclusions

Long term blockade of the thromboxane A2 receptor with GR32191B did not prevent restenosis or reduced clinical events after coronary angioplasty.

MERCATOR

Multicenter European Research Trial With Cilazapril After Angioplasty to Prevent Transluminal Coronary Obstruction and Restenosis

Title	Does the new angiotensin converting enzyme inhibitor cilazapril prevent restenosis after percutaneous transluminal coronary angioplasty? Results of the MERCATOR study: a multicenter. randomized, double-blind placebo-controlled trial.
Authors	The MERCATOR Study Group.
Reference	Circulation 1992;86:100-110.
Disease	Coronary artery disease, restenosis.
Purpose	To assess the effect of angiotensin converting enzyme inhibition with cilazapril on restenosis after coronary angioplasty.
Design	Randomized, double blind, placebo-controlled, multicenter.
Patients	693 patients with successful angioplasty of a coronary artery.
Follow-up	Clinical evaluation, exercise test, and repeated angiography at 6 months
Treatment regimen	Medications were started in the evening following the angioplasty. Cilazapril 2.5 mg PO initially, and then 5 mg X2/d or placebo for 6 months.
Additional therapy	Aspirin 150-250 mg/d, started before angioplasty. IV heparin 10,000 U bolus before angioplasty, and infusion. calcium channel blockers for 48 h were permitted.

MERCATOR

Multicenter European Research Trial With Cilazapril After Angioplasty to Prevent Transluminal Coronary Obstruction and Restenosis

(continued)

Results The mean difference in minimal coronary luminal diameter between the baseline and follow-up angiography was –0.29±0.49 and -0.27±0.51 mm in the control and cilazapril treated patients, respectively. The occurrence of clinical events including death, myocardial infarction, coronary revascularization, or recurrent angina were similar in both groups. 63.6% and 62.2% of the control and cilazapril patients were event-free after 6 months. No difference in exercise test results were found between the groups.

Conclusions Long term angiotensin converting enzyme inhibition with cilazapril did not prevent restenosis and did not reduce clinical events.

PARK

Post-Angioplasty Restenosis Ketanserin

Title	Evaluation of ketanserin in the prevention of restenosis after percutaneous transluminal coronary angioplasty. A multicenter randomized double-blind placebo-controlled trial.
Authors	Serruys PW, Klein W, Tijssen JPG, et al.
Reference	Circulation 1993;88:1588-1601.
Disease	Coronary artery disease, restenosis.
Purpose	To evaluate the role of ketanserin in prevention of restenosis after coronary angioplasty.
Design	Randomized, double blind, placebo controlled, multicenter.
Patients	658 patients, >30 years old, with angina due to a single or multivessel coronary artery disease who underwent coronary angioplasty.
Follow-up	Clinical evaluation and repeated angiography at 6 months.
Treatment regimen	Oral ketanserin 40 mg X2/d or placebo started 1 h before balloon insertion and continued for 6 months (the first 79 patients received IV infusion of ketanserin or placebo).
Additional therapy	Aspirin 250-500 mg/d, started before angioplasty. Heparin 10,000 U bolus before procedure.

Results

Clinical follow-up of 525 patients was reported. There was no difference in the occurrence of any of the clinical end points (death, myocardial infarction, coronary bypass surgery, or repeated angioplasty) between the two groups. Any of the end points occurred in 28% and 32% of the ketanserin and placebo patients (RR 0.89, 95% CI 0.70-1.13). 592 patients underwent serial angiographic studies. The mean loss of minimal luminal diameter between the post-angioplasty and follow-up angiogram was 0.27±0.49 and 0.24±0.52 mm in the ketanserin and placebo groups (difference 0.03 mm, 95% CI -0.05-0.11, p=0.5). Restenosis (>50%) occurred in 32% and 32% of the patients, respectively.

Conclusions

Ketanserin at a dose of 80 mg/d failed to reduce restenosis rate and did not lower the incidence of adverse clinical events at 6 months.

CABADAS

Prevention of Coronary Artery Bypass Graft Occlusion by Aspirin, Dipyridamole, and Acenocoumarol/Phenoprocoumon Study

Title	a. Prevention of one-year vein graft occlusion after aorto-coronary-bypass surgery: a comparison of low-dose aspirin, low-dose aspirin plus dipyridamole, and oral anti-coagulants. b. Effects of low dose aspirin (50 mg/d), low dose aspirin plus dipyridamole, and oral anticoagulant agents after internal mammary artery bypass grafting: patency and clinical outcome at 1 year.
Authors	a. van der Meer J, Hillege HL, Kootstra GJ, et al. b. van der Meer J, de la Rivière AB, van Gilst WH, et al.
Reference	a. Lancet 1993;342:257-264. b. J Am Coll Cardiol 1994;24:1181-1188.
Disease	Coronary artery disease, coronary artery bypass grafting.
Purpose	To assess the benefits of low-dose aspirin, aspirin+dipyridamole, and anticoagulation on one-year patency rate of: a. vein-grafts, b. internal thoracic artery bypass.
Design	Randomized, double blind (placebo controlled for dipyridamole, open label for anticoagulation), multicenter.
Patients	a. 948 patients, ≤70 years old, who underwent elective aortocoronary bypass surgery with saphenous vein grafts. Patients with unstable angina or myocardial infarction within 7 d were excluded. b. 494 patients of the previous group, who received both internal thoracic artery and vein grafts.
Follow-up	Clinical follow-up and coronary angiography after 1 year.

CABADAS

Prevention of Coronary Artery Bypass Graft Occlusion by Aspirin, Dipyridamole, and Acenocoumarol/Phenoprocoumon Study

(continued)

Treatment regimen

1. Aspirin 50 mg/d started after surgery.
2. Aspirin 50 mg/d started after surgery + dipyridamole IV 5 mg/kg/d started before surgery and continued for 28 h, and then orally 200 mg X2/d.
3. Oral anticoagulation, started 1 d before surgery. Target INR 2.8-4.8.

Additional therapy

Coronary artery bypass grafting surgery. Paracetamol as an analgesic. Drugs that interfere with platelet aggregation were prohibited.

Results

a. After 1 year, occlusion rate of distal anastomosis was 11% in the aspirin+dipyridamole, 15% in the aspirin alone, and 13% in the oral anticoagulation (aspirin+dipyridamole vs aspirin RR 0.76, 95% CI 0.54-1.05, oral anticoagulants vs aspirin+dipyridamole RR 0.90, 95% CI 0.65-1.25). Clinical events (death, myocardial infarction, thrombosis, or major bleeding) occurred in 20.3%, 13.9% (RR 1.46, 95% CI 1.02-2.08), and 16.9% (RR 1.22, 95% CI 0.84-1.77), respectively.
b. Occlusion rates were 4.6%, 5.3%, and 6.8% in the aspirin+dipyridamole, aspirin, and oral anticoagulants (p=NS). Overall clinical event rates were 23.3%, 13.3% (RR 1.75, 95% CI 1.09-2.81, p=0.025), and 17.1% (RR 1.29, 95% CI 0.77-2.15, p=0.42), respectively.

Conclusions

Addition of dipyridamole to low-dose aspirin did not improve patency of either venous or internal thoracic artery grafts significantly. However, the overall clinical event rate was increased by adding dipyridamole.

EPIC

Evaluation of 7E3 for the Prevention of Ischemic Complications

Title	a. Randomized trial of coronary intervention with antibody against platelet IIb/IIIa integrin for reduction of clinical restenosis: results at six months. b. Use of monoclonal antibody directed against the platelet glycoprotein IIb/IIIa receptor in high-risk coronary angioplasty.
Authors	a. Topol EJ, Califf RM, Weisman HF, et al. b. The EPIC Investigators.
Reference	a. Lancet 1994;343:881-886. b. N Engl J Med 1994;330:956-961.
Disease	Coronary artery disease, restenosis.
Purpose	To evaluate the effect of a monoclonal antibody Fab fragment (c7E3), directed against the IIb/IIIa integrin, to reduce restenosis following balloon angioplasty or directional atherectomy of coronary lesions in high risk coronary lesions.
Design	Randomized, double blind, placebo controlled, multicenter.
Patients	2099 patients, age <80 years, who needed coronary angioplasty or directional atherectomy and had an evolving or recent myocardial infarction, unstable angina, or high risk angiographic or clinical characteristics.
Follow-up	6 month clinical follow-up.
Treatment regimen	1. Placebo bolus and placebo infusion for 12 h; 2. c7E3 0.25 mg/kg bolus and placebo infusion for 12 h; and 3. c7E3 0.25 mg/kg bolus and 10 μg/min infusion for 12 h. The bolus was given at least 10 min before procedure.

Additional therapy

Aspirin 325 mg/d, with the first dose at least 2 h before procedure. IV heparin bolus 10,000-12,000 U before procedure and for ≥12 h after the procedure.

Results

Bleeding complications that mandated transfusion occurred in 7%, 14%, and 17% of the 3 groups, respectively ($p<0.001$). There was no difference in the events rates during the first 48 h. At 30 days, the composite end point of death, infarction, and repeated revascularization occurred in 12.8%, 11.5%, and 8.3%, respectively (c7E3 bolus+infusion vs placebo $p=0.008$). >48 h-6 months, the composite end point occurred in 25.4%, 24.3%, and 19.2%, respectively ($p=0.007$). Total events rates within 6 months were 35.1%, 32.6%, and 27.0%, respectively ($p=0.001$). The favorable long-term effect was mainly due to reduced need for repeated revascularization (22.3%, 21.0%, and 16.5%, respectively ($p=0.007$). By regression analysis the c7E3 bolus+infusion was independently associated with fewer events during the 6 month follow-up (hazard ratio 0.75, $p=0.025$).

Conclusions

c7E3 bolus and infusion reduced the revascularization procedure rate during 6 month follow-up of high-risk angioplasty patients. However, bleeding complications were increased.

ERA

Enoxaparin Restenosis Trial

Title	Low molecular weight heparin in prevention of restenosis after angioplasty. Results of enoxaparin restenosis (ERA) trial.
Authors	Faxon DP, Spiro TE, Minor S, et al.
Reference	Circulation 1994;90:908-914.
Disease	Coronary artery disease, restenosis.
Purpose	To evaluate whether enoxaparin given subcutaneously for 28 days will reduce the restenosis rates after coronary angioplasty.
Design	Randomized, double blind, placebo controlled, multicenter.
Patients	458 patients, >21 years old, with ≥50% stenosis of a coronary artery, reduced to <50% with ≥20% change in diameter by angioplasty. Patients with asthma, hypertension, acute myocardial infarction within 5 days, angioplasty of venous grafts, or restenosis after prior angioplasty were excluded.
Follow-up	Clinical evaluation, exercise test, and repeated angiography at 24 weeks.
Treatment regimen	Enoxaparin 40 mg/d SC or placebo, started <24 h after angioplasty and continued for 28 d.
Additional therapy	Aspirin 325 mg/d started 1 d before procedure. IV heparin was given during angioplasty. calcium channel blockers before and after angioplasty.

Results

Restenosis (loss of >50% of the initial gain in luminal diameter or death, reinfarction, need for bypass surgery, or worsening of angina in patients without follow-up angiography) occurred in 51% of the placebo and 52% of the enoxaparin patients (RR 1.07, p=0.63). Restenosis occurred in 49% and 50% of the patients with follow-up angiography, respectively. The late loss of minimal luminal diameter was 0.49 and 0.54 mm, in the control and enoxaparin, respectively (p=0.78). Adverse clinical events were infrequent and similar between the groups. Minor bleeding complications were more common with enoxaparin (48% vs 34%). In a subset of patients, there was no difference in performance in exercise test.

Conclusions

Enoxaparin 40 mg/d did not reduce the occurrence of restenosis or of adverse clinical events.

MARCATOR

Multicenter American Research Trial With Cilazapril After Angioplasty to Prevent Transluminal Coronary Obstruction and Restenosis

Title	Effect of high dose angiotensin-converting enzyme inhibition on restenosis: final results of the MARCATOR study, a multicenter, double blind, placebo-controlled trial of cilazapril.
Authors	Faxon DP, MARCATOR Study Group.
Reference	J Am Coll Cardiol 1995;25:362-369.
Disease	Coronary artery disease, restenosis.
Purpose	To assess the effect of high and low dose angiotensin converting enzyme inhibition on restenosis after coronary angioplasty.
Design	Randomized, double blind, placebo-controlled, multicenter.
Patients	1436 patients, age 25-80 years, without recent myocardial infarction (<5 days), prior revascularization, or severe hypertension or valvular disease.
Follow-up	Clinical evaluation and repeated angiography at 24 weeks.
Treatment regimen	Study medication were started <6 h after successful angioplasty and continued for 6 months. 1. Cilazapril 1mg X2/d 2. Cilazapril 5 mg X2/d. 3. Cilazapril 10 mg X2/d. 4. Placebo.
Additional therapy	Aspirin 325 mg/d, started before angioplasty. IV heparin 10,000 U before procedure, and infusion thereafter. calcium channel blockers were recommended.

MARCATOR

Multicenter American Research Trial With Cilazapril After Angioplasty to Prevent Transluminal Coronary Obstruction and Restenosis

(continued)

Results

The mean difference in minimal coronary lumen diameter between the baseline and follow-up angiography was -0.35±0.51, -0.37±0.52, -0.45±0.52, and -0.41±0.53 mm for the placebo, 2, 10, and 20 mg/d cilazapril, respectively (p=NS). Restenosis >50% at follow-up occurred in 33%, 40%, 36%, and 34%, respectively. Clinical events during follow-up did not differ among the 4 groups.

Conclusions

Long term angiotensin-converting enzyme inhibition with cilazapril did not prevent restenosis and did not reduce clinical event rate after angioplasty.

SHARP

The Subcutaneous Heparin and Angioplasty Restenosis Prevention (SHARP) Trial

Title	The Subcutaneous Heparin and Angioplasty Restenosis Prevention (SHARP) Trial. Results of a multicenter randomized trial investigating the effects of high dose unfractionated heparin on angiographic restenosis and clinical outcome.
Authors	Brack MJ, Ray S, Chauhan A, et al.
Reference	J Am Coll Cardiol 1995;26:947-954.
Disease	Coronary artery disease.
Purpose	To investigate whether high dose subcutaneous heparin will improve outcome after coronary angioplasty.
Design	Randomized, open label with blinded analysis of data, three centers.
Patients	339 patients who had undergone successful coronary angioplasty. Patients with restenotic lesions, chronic total occlusions or conduit lesions were not included.
Follow-up	4 month clinical evaluation and repeated angiography.
Treatment regimen	Subcutaneous heparin 12,500 U X2/d for 4 months, started 2 h after femoral sheath removal, or no therapy.
Additional therapy	Coronary angioplasty, aspirin 300 mg and heparin IV bolus 10,000 U before the procedure. After angioplasty, heparin infusion 1,000 U/h for up to 24 h. Aspirin 75-300 mg/d. Other medications according to operator choice.

SHARP

The Subcutaneous Heparin and Angioplasty Restenosis Prevention (SHARP) Trial

(continued)

Results

Repeated angiography was performed in 90% of the patients. The difference in minimal luminal diameter between the post-angioplasty and follow-up study was -0.55±0.58 mm for the control and -0.43±0.59 mm for the heparin group (p=NS). The occurrence of myocardial infarction, coronary artery bypass surgery, repeated angioplasty, and angina at 4 months was comparable. There was no difference between the groups in the number of patients with ischemia during follow-up exercise test.

Conclusions

Long term treatment with high dose subcutaneous heparin for 4 months failed to improve outcome and to prevent restenosis.

REDUCE

Reviparin in percutaneous transluminal coronary angioplasty

Title	Low molecular weight heparin (Reviparin) in percutaneous transluminal coronary angioplasty. Results of a randomized, double-blind, unfractionated heparin and placebo-controlled, multicenter trial (REDUCE trial).
Authors	Karsch KR, Preisack MB, Baildon R, et al.
Reference	J Am Coll Cardiol 1996;28:1437-1443.
Disease	Coronary artery disease.
Purpose	To evaluate the effect of low molecular weight heparin on the incidence of restenosis in patients with coronary artery disease undergoing percutaneous transluminal coronary angioplasty (PTCA).
Design	Randomized, double blind, multicenter.
Patients	612 patients with single-lesion coronary artery obstruction scheduled to undergo coronary angioplasty. Patients with class 3C unstable angina or unstable angina requiring continuous heparin infusion, myocardial infarction within 14 days, bleeding disorders, active peptic ulcer, uncontrolled asthma or hypertension, left main coronary artery stenosis >50%, and angioplasty of saphenous vein graft or previous angioplasty at the same site were excluded.
Follow-up	Clinical follow-up for 30 weeks. Repeated coronary angiography at 26±2 weeks after angioplasty.

REDUCE

Reviparin in percutaneous transluminal coronary angioplasty

(continued)

Treatment regimen

At the time of arterial access, patients were randomized to either a bolus of unfractionated heparin (10,000 IU), followed by infusion of 24,000 IU heparin over 16±4h, or reviparin (7,000 IU anti-Xa U), followed by infusion of reviparin 10,500 IU anti-Xa U over 16±4h. Then, patients received either 3,500 IU anti-Xa U of reviparin or placebo subcutaneously X2/d for 28 days.

Additional therapy

Standard balloon angioplasty. Aspirin 100 mg/d was started one day before angioplasty.

Results

By intention to treat analysis, treatment failure (death, myocardial infarction, bypass surgery, or emergency or elective repeat angioplasty) occurred in 33.3% of the reviparin and 32.0% of the controls (p=0.71). Angiographic restenosis was present in 33.0% of patients of the reviparin vs 34.4% of the control group. 16.4% of the reviparin vs 19.9% of the control group developed significant angina. Acute events within 24 hours after the procedure occurred less often in the reviparin-treated group (3.9% vs 8.2%, respectively; relative risk (RR) 0.49; 95% CI 0.26-0.92; p=0.027). Only 6 patients in the reviparin-treated group vs 21 patients in the control group needed emergency stent implantation (RR 0.29; 95% CI 0.13-0.66; p=0.003). Analysis of primary end-points after 30 weeks revealed that the occurrence of clinical events was comparable between the groups (31.7% vs 30% in the reviparin and control, respectively). There was no difference in late loss of minimal lumen diameter between the two groups. Bleeding complications were comparable (2.3% in the reviparin vs 2.6% in the control group; p=0.8).

Conclusions

Reviparin use started immediately before coronary balloon angioplasty and continued for 28 days did not reduce the rate of major clinical events or the incidence of restenosis over 30 weeks follow-up.

ISAR

Intracoronary Stenting and Antithrombotic Regimen trial

Title	A randomized comparison of antiplatelets and anticoagulant therapy after the placement of coronary-artery stents.
Authors	Schömig A, Neumann F-J, Kastrati A, et al.
Reference	N Engl J Med 1996;334:1084-1089.
Disease	Coronary artery disease, restenosis.
Purpose	To compare the efficacy of two therapeutic regimens after placement of coronary artery stents: 1. combined antiplatelet therapy with ticlopidine plus aspirin, and 2. anticoagulation with intravenous heparin, phenprocoumon, and aspirin.
Design	Randomized, one center.
Patients	257 patients in whom intracoronary Palmaz-Schatz stents were successfully implanted after balloon angioplasty. The indications for stenting were extensive dissection after angioplasty, complete vessel closure, residual stenosis ≥30%, and lesions in venous bypass grafts. Patients with absolute indication for anticoagulation, or contraindications to one of the drugs, cardiogenic shock, or who had needed mechanical ventilation were excluded.
Follow-up	Hospitalization for 10 days. Clinical follow-up for 30 days.
Treatment regimen	In patients assigned to antiplatelet therapy, heparin infusion was started after arterial sheath removal for 12 h. Ticlopidine 250 mgX2/d was administered for 4 weeks. In patients assigned to anticoagulation therapy, heparin infusion, started after sheath removal, was continued for 5 to 10 days. Phenoprocoumon was given for 4 weeks (target INR 3.5 to 4.5).

ISAR

Intracoronary Stenting and Antithrombotic Regimen trial

(continued)

Additional therapy	Heparin and aspirin intravenously before PTCA. All patients received aspirin 100 mgX2/d throughout the study.
Results	30 days after randomization, mortality was comparable (0.4% vs 0.8% in the antiplatelet and anticoagulant group, respectively). Myocardial infarction occurred in 0.8% vs 4.2% of the patients, respectively (relative risk (RR) 0.18; 95% CI 0.02 to 0.83; p=0.02), and the need for revascularization was 1.2% vs 5.4% (RR 0.22; 95% CI 0.04 to 0.77; p=0.01). A primary cardiac event (cardiac death, myocardial infarction, or revascularization) occurred in 1.6% of the antiplatelet vs 6.2% of the anticoagulant patients (RR 0.25; 95% CI 0.06 to 0.77; p=0.01). Occlusion of the stented vessel occurred less often in the antiplatelet group (0.8% vs 5.4%; RR 0.14; 95% CI 0.02 to 0.62; p=0.004). A primary non-cardiac endpoint (non-cardiac death, cerebrovascular accident, or severe peripheral vascular or hemorrhagic event) was reached by 1.2% vs 12.3% of the antiplatelet and anticoagulant groups, respectively (RR 0.09; 95% CI 0.02 to 0.31; p<0.001). Bleeding complications occurred only in the anticoagulant group (6.5%; p<0.001). Peripheral vascular events occurred in 0.8% of the antiplatelet group vs 6.2% of the anticoagulant group (RR 0.13; 95% CI 0.01 to 0.53; p=0.001).
Conclusions	After successful placement of coronary artery stents, the combination of aspirin and ticlopidine was associated with lower rate of cardiac events and fewer vascular and hemorrhagic complications.

ACCORD

Angioplasie Coronaire Corvasal Diltiazem

Title	Effect of the direct nitric oxide donors linsidomine and molsidomine on angiographic restenosis after coronary balloon angioplasty. The ACCORD study.
Authors	Lablanche J-M, Grollier G, Lusson J-R, et al.
Reference	Circulation 1997;95:83-89
Disease	Coronary artery disease, restenosis.
Purpose	To evaluate the effect of molsidomine and linsidomine, direct nitric oxide donors, on restenosis after coronary balloon angioplasty.
Design	Randomized, multicenter.
Patients	700 patients, ≤70 years old, with angina and/or evidence of myocardial ischemia who were referred for balloon angioplasty. Patients with myocardial infarction within 3 months, recent unstable angina, ejection fraction <0.35, systolic blood pressure <100 mmHg, contraindications to aspirin, restenotic graft or left main coronary artery lesions and totally occluded lesions were excluded.
Follow-up	Clinical follow-up with repeated coronary angiography at 6 months.
Treatment regimen	Randomization to active treatment group or controls. The active treatment consisted of continuous infusion of linsidomine (1 mg/h), started 3 to 18 h before the angioplasty, and continued for 24 h after the procedure, and then, molsidomine 4mgX3/d PO for 6 months. The control group received diltiazem 60 mgX3/d.

Additional therapy

Aspirin 250 mg/d. Heparin 10,000 IU at the start of angioplasty, additional doses of heparin 5000 IU after each hour of procedure. Long-acting nitrates, calcium channel blockers, oral anticoagulants, and angiotensin converting enzyme inhibitors were prohibited.

Results

520 patients had three angiograms (at baseline, immediately after angioplasty, and at follow-up). Despite the intracoronary administration of isosorbide dinitrate before angiography, the mean reference luminal diameter was greater in the NO donor group than in the diltiazem group before angioplasty (2.94 vs 2.83 mm; p=0.014). The mean minimal luminal diameter (MLD) before angioplasty was comparable. However, immediately after angioplasty, MLD was 1.94 vs 1.81 mm, in the NO donor and the diltiazem group, respectively; p=0.001). Mean MLD remained larger in the NO donor group at follow-up (1.54 vs 1.38 mm; p=0.007). Late loss, loss index, and the slope of the regression between late loss and acute gain were comparable. At 6 months, restenosis (≥50%) occurred in 38.0% of the NO donor treated patients vs 46.5% of the diltiazem group (p=0.062). After adjustment for center and hypercholesterolemia the p value was 0.026. The combined rate of major clinical events (death, myocardial infarction, and coronary revascularization) were comparable (32.2% in the NO donor group vs 32.4% in the diltiazem group). The incidence of side effects and the number of dropouts due to adverse effects were similar (13 vs 10, respectively).

Conclusions

NO donor therapy was associated with larger MLD immediately after and at follow-up following coronary balloon angioplasty and lower rate of restenosis. However, late luminal loss did not differ between the groups and there was no difference in the occurrence of major clinical events.

5. Hypertension

SHEP

Systolic Hypertension in the Elderly Program

Title	Prevention of stroke by antihypertensive drug treatment in older persons with isolated systolic hypertension. Final results of the systolic hypertension in the elderly program (SHEP).
Authors	SHEP Cooperative Research Group.
Reference	JAMA 1991;265:3255-3264.
Disease	Hypertension.
Purpose	To evaluate the efficacy of antihypertensive drug therapy to reduce the risk of stroke in patients with isolated systolic hypertension.
Design	Randomized, double blind, placebo controlled, multicenter.
Patients	4736 patients, ≥60 years old, with systolic blood pressure 160-219, and diastolic blood pressure <90 mm Hg. Patients with major cardiovascular diseases or other serious illnesses were excluded.
Follow-up	Average 4.5 years.
Treatment regimen	The goal of blood pressure reduction was <160 mmHg systolic blood pressure for those with initial pressure >180 mmHg, and by at least 20 mmHg for those with initial pressure 160-179 mmHg. Patients were randomized to placebo or chlorthalidone 12.5 mg/d. Dose was doubled if the pressure goal was not reached, and then atenolol 25 mg/d or placebo was added. If contraindications existed, reserpine 0.05 mg/d was given.
Additional therapy	Potassium supplements to all patients with serum K <3.5 mmol/l.

SHEP

Systolic Hypertension in the Elderly Program

(continued)

Results

After 5 years 44% of the placebo group received active antihypertensive therapy. During the trial, the goal blood pressure was reached by 65%-72% of the active drug therapy vs 32%-40% of the placebo group. Mean systolic blood pressure was lower in the active treatment than the placebo group throughout the protocol. By life table analysis, 5-year cumulative stroke rates were 5.2% vs 8.2% for the active therapy and placebo groups, respectively (RR 0.64, 95% CI 0.50-0.82, p=0.0003). After a mean of 4.5 years follow-up the mortality was 9.0% vs 10.2% (RR 0.87 (0.73-1.05)), myocardial infarction occurred in 2.1% vs 3.1% (RR 0.67 (0.47-0.96)), left ventricular failure in 2.0% vs 4.3% (RR 0.46 (0.33-0.65)), and total major cardiovascular events in 12.2% vs 17.5% (RR 0.68 (0.58-0.79)).

Conclusions

Stepped-care drug therapy for isolated systolic hypertension in patients ≥60 years old reduced the incidence of major cardiovascular events and stroke.

TOMHS

Treatment of Mild Hypertension Study

Title	a. Characteristics of participants in the treatment of mild hypertension study (TOMHS). b. The treatment of mild hypertension study. A randomized, placebo-controlled trial of a nutritional-hygienic regimen along with various drug monotherapies. c. Treatment of mild hypertension study. Final results.
Authors	a. Masciolo SR, Grimm RH, Neaton JD, et al. b. TOMHS Research Group. c. Neaton JD, Grimm RH Jr, Prineas RJ, et al.
Reference	a. Am J Cardiol 1990;66:32C-35C. b. Arch Intern Med 1991;151:1413-1423. c. JAMA 1993;270:713-724.
Disease	Hypertension.
Purpose	To assess the relative efficacy and safety of a non-pharmacological therapy alone with those of non-pharmacological therapy and 5 pharmacological monotherapy regimens.
Design	Randomized, double blind, multicenter.
Patients	902 patients, age 45-69 years, with mild hypertension (diastolic blood pressure 90-99 mmHg, or if they were previously treated with antihypertensive drugs, 85-99 mmHg). Patients with cardiovascular disease or life-threatening illness were excluded.
Follow-up	>4 years (mean 4.4 years).

TOMHS

Treatment of Mild Hypertension Study

(continued)

Treatment regimen	Randomization to: 1. acebutalol 400 mg/d; 2. amlodipine 5 mg/d; 3. chlorthalidone 15 mg/d; 4. doxazosin 1 mg/d for 1 month and then 2 mg/d; 5. enalapril 5 mg/d; 6. placebo. For a participant with diastolic blood pressure ≥95 mmHg on 3 visits, or ≥105 mmHg at a single visit, medication dose was doubled. If blood pressure remained high, a second drug was added. For all groups, except the diuretic group, chlorothalidone 15 mg/d was added. In the chlorthalidone group, enalapril 2.5 mg was given.
Additional therapy	Behavior change, 10% weight loss, lowering sodium intake to ≤70 mmol/d, lowering alcohol intake, and increasing activity.
Results	After 12 months, weight loss averaged 4.5 kg, urinary sodium excretion declined by 23%, and physical activity was almost doubled. After 12 months blood pressure was decreased by 20.1±1.4/13.7±0.7, 17.5±1.1/12.9±0.7, 21.8±1.3/13.1±0.7, 16.1±1.2/ 12.0±0.7, 17.6±1.2/12.2±0.7, and 10.6±1.0/8.1±0.5 mmHg in groups 1-6, respectively (P<0.01 for each drug compared to placebo). Overall the compliance and tolerance were good for all groups and side effects were acceptable. After 4 years, 59% of the placebo and 72% of the active drug groups continued their initial drug as monotherapy. Major clinical events occurred in 7.3% of the placebo vs 5.1% of the active drug groups (p=0.21), and major cardiovascular event in 5.1% vs 3.9%, respectively (p=0.42). Average decrease in LV mass was 24, 25, 34, 24, 23, and 27 grams for groups 1-6. The only significant difference vs placebo for reduction in LV mass was with chlorthalidone (p=0.03).
Conclusions	Adding one of the five different classes of drugs resulted in significant additional decrease of blood pressure with minimal side effects. Differences among the five drug groups did not consistently favor one over the others concerning regression of left ventricular mass, blood lipid levels, and other clinical outcomes.

STOP-Hypertension

Swedish Trial in Old Patients With Hypertension

Title	a. Morbidity and mortality in the Swedish Trial in Old Patients with Hypertension (STOP-Hypertension). b. Swedish trial in old patients with hypertension (STOP-Hypertension). Analyses performed up to 1992.
Authors	Dahlöf B, Lindholm LH, Hansson L, et al.
Reference	a. Lancet 1991;338:1281-1285. b. Clin Exper Hypertension 1993;15:925-939.
Disease	Hypertension.
Purpose	To evaluate the efficacy of pharmacological treatment of hypertension in patients 70-84 years old.
Design	Randomized, double blind, placebo controlled, multicenter.
Patients	1627 patients, age 70-84 years, with blood pressure ≥180/90 mmHg, or diastolic blood pressure >105 mmHg. Patients with blood pressure above 230/120 mmHg, orthostatic hypotension, or myocardial infarction or stroke within the previous 12 months were excluded.
Follow-up	1-4 years (average of 25 months).
Treatment regimen	Patients were randomized to either active therapy or placebo. The centers were free to chose one of the 4 following agents: Atenolol 50 mg/d, hydrochlorothiazide 25 mg/d + amiloride 2.5 mg/d, metoprolol 100 mg/d, or pindolol 5 mg/d. If blood pressure was >160/95 mmHg after 2 months of therapy, diuretic therapy was added to the ß blocker, and vice versa. If blood pressure exceeded 230/120 mmHg on two subsequent visits, open antihypertensive therapy was given.

STOP-Hypertension

Swedish Trial in Old Patients With Hypertension

(continued)

Results

a. Compared with placebo, active therapy reduced the number of myocardial infarctions (16.5 vs 14.4 per 1000 patient-years, RR 0.87, 95% CI 0.49-1.56), stroke (31.3 vs 16.8 per 1000 patient-years, RR 0.53, 95% CI 0.33-0.86, p=0.0081), total mortality (35.4 vs 20.2 per 1000 patient-years, RR 0.57, 95% CI 0.37-0.87, p=0.0079), and the occurrence of the primary endpoints (stroke, myocardial infarction or cardiovascular death) (55.5 vs 33.5 per 1000 patient-years, RR 0.60, 95% CI 0.43-0.85, p=0.0031).
b. A majority of the patients needed combined treatment to reach the goal blood pressure (160/95 mmHg). The impact on mortality and morbidity was greater than previously seen in middle-aged patients. Women benefited from treatment at least as much as men.

Conclusions

Antihypertensive therapy in hypertensive patients aged 70-84 reduced cardiovascular morbidity and mortality.

TAIM

Trial of Antihypertensive Interventions and Management

Title

a. Effect of drug and diet treatment of mild hypertension on diastolic blood pressure.
b. The Trial of Antihypertensive Interventions and Management (TAIM) study. Adequate weight loss, alone and combined with drug therapy in the treatment of mild hypertension.
c. Effect of antihypertensives on sexual function and quality of life: the TAIM study.

Authors

a. Langford HG, Davis BR, Blaufox D, et al.
b. Wassertheil-Smoller S, Blaufox MD, Oberman AS, et al.
c. Wassertheil-Smoller S, Blaufox D, Oberman A, et al.

Reference

a. Hypertension 1991;17:210-217.
b. Arch Intern Med 1992;152:131-136.
c. Ann Intern Med 1991;114:613-620.

Disease

Hypertension.

Purpose

To evaluate the relative efficacy of various combinations of the commonly used approaches to drug and diet therapy for hypertension.

Design

Randomized, double blind (drug therapy), placebo controlled, 3X3 factorial, three centers.

Patients

787 patients, age 21-65 years, with diastolic blood pressure 90-100 mmHg without medications, and body weight of 110-160% of the ideal body weight. Patients with prior stroke, myocardial infarction, asthma, insulin treated diabetes mellitus, and renal failure were excluded.

Follow-up

6 months.

Treatment regimen

Nine groups of treatment combinations of one out of three drug regimens with one out of three diet interventions. The drugs were: placebo, chlorthalidone 25 mg, or atenolol 50 mg. The diet interventions were: usual, a weight reduction (goal 10% of basal body weight or 4.54 kg), or low in sodium (52-

100 mmol/d) and high in potassium (62-115 mmol/d) diets. Patients who failed to achieve blood pressure control were given additional therapy in a double blind fashion (chlorthalidone or atenolol for the placebo and combination of atenolol and chlorthalidone to the other 2 drug groups. If diastolic blood pressure remained ≥100 mmHg, the doses were increased, and if it did not help open-label therapy was added.

Results

a. Among the placebo drug-assigned patients 20.0%, 10.0%, and 16.5% of the usual, weight loss, and low sodium diet received additional medications to control blood pressure over the 6 months of follow-up. Only 2.7% and 3.0% of the chlorthalidone and atenolol treated patients needed an additional medication. The mean weight reduction in the weight loss diet group was 4.7 kg. The low Na/high K group had an average decrease in urinary sodium of 27.4 mmol/d and increase of potassium excretion of 10.9 mmol/d. The mean reduction of diastolic blood pressure in patients on usual diet was 7.96, 10.78, and 12.43 mmHg for placebo, chlorthalidone and atenolol groups. For patients in the weight loss diet it was 8.78, 15.06 and 14.81 mmHg, respectively, and for the low Na/high K diet it was 7.91, 12.18 and 12.76 mmHg, respectively. Atenolol as a single therapy achieved the greatest reduction of blood pressure ($p=0.001$ vs low Na/high K diet alone, and $p=0.006$ vs weight loss alone. Adding weight loss diet to chlorthalidone enhanced the blood pressure lowering response significantly ($p=0.002$).
b. Among the patients assigned to placebo drug and weight loss diet, diastolic blood pressure reduction after 6 months was greater among patients who lost ≥4.5 kg than among those who achieved only <2.25 kg reduction (11.6 vs 7.0 mmHg; $p<0.046$). The effect of ≥4.5 kg body weight reduction was comparable to that of chlorthalidone or atenolol. The weight loss diet benefited quality of life most, reducing total physical complaints ($p<0.001$), and increasing satisfaction with health ($p<0.001$). Low-dose chlorthalidone and atenolol produced few side effects, except in men. Sexual problems developed in 29%, 13% and 3% of men receiving usual diet and chlorthalidone, atenolol and placebo, respectively ($p=0.006$ for the difference among groups). The low Na/high K diet was associated with increased fatigue.

Conclusions

Drug therapy was more efficient than diet intervention in reducing diastolic blood pressure. Weight loss of ≥4.5 kg is beneficial, especially in combination with diuretics.

TOHP-1

Trial of Hypertension Prevention (Phase I)

Title	a. The effects of nonpharmacologic interventions on blood pressure of persons with high normal levels. Results of the trials of hypertension prevention, phase I. b. The effect of potassium supplementation in persons with a high-normal blood pressure. results from phase I of the Trials of Hypertension Prevention (TOHP). c. Lack of blood pressure effect with calcium and magnesium supplementation in adults with high-normal blood pressure. results from phase I of the Trials of Hypertension Prevention (TOHP).
Authors	a. The Trials of Hypertension Prevention Collaborative Research Group. b. Whelton PK, Buring J, Borhani NO, et al. c. Yamamoto ME, Applegate WB, Klag MJ, et al.
Reference	a. JAMA 1992;267:1213-1220. b. Ann Epidemiol 1995;5:85-95. c. Ann Epidemiol 1995;5:96-107.
Disease	Hypertension.
Purpose	To evaluate the short-term feasibility and efficacy of seven nonpharmacologic interventions to reduce diastolic blood pressure.
Design	Three randomized, parallel-group trials, multicenter.
Patients	2182 patients, 30-54 years old, with diastolic blood pressure of 80-89 mmHg, who were not taking medications in the prior 2 months.
Follow-up	18 months.

TOHP-1

Trial of Hypertension Prevention (Phase I)

(continued)

Treatment regimen

Three life-style change groups (weight reduction, sodium intake reduction, and stress management) were each compared with unmasked nonintervention control over 18 months. 4 nutritional supplement groups (calcium, magnesium, potassium, and fish oil) were each compared in a double blind fashion with placebo controls over 6 months.

Results

Weight reduction intervention resulted in 3.9 kg weight loss ($p<0.01$, compared to baseline), diastolic blood pressure reduction of 2.3 mmHg ($p<0.01$), and systolic blood pressure reduction of 2.9 mmHg ($p<0.01$). sodium restriction intervention resulted in 44 mmol/24 h decrease of urinary sodium excretion ($p<0.01$), diastolic and systolic blood pressure reduction of 0.9 ($p<0.05$) and 1.7 mmHg ($p<0.01$). Potassium supplementation resulted in 1.8 mmHg ($p=0.04$) reduction in diastolic blood pressure after 3 months. However, the effect disappeared after 6 months (mean reduction 0.3 mmHg). Neither stress management nor nutritional supplements reduced blood pressure significantly.

Conclusions

Weight reduction was the most effective of the strategies in reducing blood pressure in normotensive persons. sodium restriction was also effective.

MRC

Medical Research Council Trial of Treatment of Hypertension in Older Adults

Title	Medical Research Council trial of treatment of hypertension in older adults: principal results.
Authors	MRC Working Party.
Reference	Br Med J 1992;304:405-412.
Disease	Hypertension.
Purpose	To evaluate the efficacy of ß blockers and diuretic therapy to reduce cardiovascular mortality and morbidity in hypertensive older adults.
Design	Randomized, single blind, placebo controlled, multicenter.
Patients	4396 patients, age 65-74 years, with systolic blood pressure 160-209 mmHg, and diastolic blood pressure <115 mmHg. Patients on antihypertensive medications, or with secondary hypertension, heart failure, angina pectoris, myocardial infarction or stroke within 3 months, impaired renal function, diabetes mellitus, asthma, or other serious intercurrent disease were excluded.
Follow-up	Mean follow-up 5.8 years (25,355 patients-years of observation).
Treatment regimen	1. Amiloride 2.5 mg/d+ hydrochlorothiazide 25 mg/d or placebo. 2. Atenolol 50 mg/d or placebo. Drug doses were modified to reach the target blood pressure of 150-160 mmHg.
Additional therapy	Additional therapy was started if mean blood pressure was >115 mmHg, or systolic blood pressure >210 mmHg.

Medical Research Council Trial of Treatment of Hypertension in Older Adults

(continued)

Results

Both treatment arms reduced systolic blood pressure compared with the placebo group. After 3 months, the diuretic therapy reduced blood pressure more than atenolol. However, after 2 years, systolic and diastolic blood pressures were similar in the diuretics and atenolol groups. More patients randomized to atenolol required supplementary drugs to control hypertension than the diuretic group (52% vs 38%). The atenolol group had significantly more withdrawals from the study compared to diuretics for both suspected major side effects and inadequate blood pressure control (345 vs 161 patients, respectively). In the placebo group 257 patients were withdrawn. The number of strokes was reduced with active therapy (7.3%, 9.0% and 10.8% in the diuretics, atenolol, and placebo groups (25% reduction of risk (active therapy vs placebo), 95% CI 3-42%, p=0.04). Coronary events occurred in 7.7%, 12.8%, and 12.7%, respectively (19% reduction of risk (active therapy vs placebo), 95% CI -2% to 36%, p=0.08). Total mortality was not different among the groups (21.3%, 26.4% and 24.7%, respectively). After adjusting for baseline characteristics the diuretic group had reduced risks of stroke (31%, 95% CI 3%-51%, p=0.04), coronary events (44%, 95% CI 21%-60%, p=0.0009), and all cardiovascular events (35%, 95% CI 17%-49%, p=0.0005), compared with placebo. The atenolol group showed no significant reduction in these end points. Reduction of stroke was mainly in non-smokers taking diuretics.

Conclusions

Hydrochlorothiazide and amiloride are better than atenolol in reducing the incidence of stroke and coronary events in older hypertensive patients.

Metoprolol in the Treatment of Hypertension in the Elderly

Title	Safety and efficacy of metoprolol in the treatment of hypertension in the elderly.
Authors	LaPalio L, Schork A, Glasser S, Tifft C.
Reference	J Am Geriatr Soc 1992;40:354-358.
Disease	Hypertension.
Purpose	To evaluate the short-term efficacy and safety of metoprolol in the treatment of hypertension in patients 50-75 years old.
Design	Open label, surveillance, multicenter.
Patients	21,692 patients, 50-75 years old, with hypertension (systolic blood pressure ≤200 mmHg and diastolic blood pressure 90-104 mmHg for patients that had not been under therapy before and ≤95 mmHg for those who were previously treated). Patients who needed β blockers for angina, patients with heart block or bradycardia <55 bpm, congestive heart failure, or intolerance to β blockers were excluded.
Follow-up	8 week clinical follow-up.
Treatment regimen	Metoprolol 100 mg/d. If diastolic blood pressure remained >90 mmHg after 4 weeks, hydrochlorothiazide 25 mg/d was added.

Results After 4 weeks mean systolic and diastolic blood pressure were reduced from 162/95 to 148/87 mmHg ($p<0.001$). 58% of the patients had adequate blood pressure control with 100 mg/d metoprolol. After 8 weeks blood pressure decreased to 143/84 mmHg. At the termination of the study 50% of the patients continued with metoprolol as monotherapy, and 27% needed combined therapy. There was <5% incidence of medical problems. Excellent or good tolerability was noted for 94% of the patients.

Conclusions Metoprolol administered either as monotherapy or in combination with diuretic was an effective and safe therapy for elderly hypertensive patients.

Veterans Affairs Cooperative Study Group on Antihypertensive Agents

Title	Single-drug therapy for hypertension in men. A comparison of six antihypertensive agents with placebo.
Authors	Materson BJ, Reda DJ, Cushman WC, et al.
Reference	N Engl J Med 1993;328:914-921.
Disease	Hypertension.
Purpose	To compare the efficacy of different classes of antihypertensive agents as monotherapy for hypertension according to age and race.
Design	Randomized, double blind, placebo controlled, multicenter.
Patients	1292 men, age ≥21 years, and diastolic blood pressure 95-109 mmHg on placebo.
Follow-up	For at least 1 year.
Treatment regimen	Randomization to: 1. placebo; 2. hydrochlorothiazide 12.5-50 mg/d; 3. atenolol 25-100 mg/d; 4. clonidine 0.2-0.6 mg/d; 5. captopril 25-100 mg/d; 6. prazosin 4-20 mg/d; and 7. sustained-release diltiazem 120-360 mg/d. Patients who reached diastolic blood pressure <90 mmHg on 2 visits entered a maintenance phase for ≥1 year.

Results

At the end of the titration phase 33%, 57%, 65%, 65%, 54%, 56%, and 75% of the patients in groups 1-7 reached diastolic blood pressure <90 mmHg. 745 patients reached diastolic blood pressure <90 mmHg without intolerable side effects during the titration phase and entered the maintenance phase. The percentage of patients with initial control of blood pressure in whom diastolic blood pressure remained <95 mmHg over 1 year was similar among groups (p=0.93). However, by intention to treat analysis, 25%, 46%, 51%, 50%, 42%, 42%, and 59% of the patients in groups 1-7 had reached diastolic blood pressure <90 mmHg during the titration phase and <95 mmHg during the maintenance phase (p<0.001 for a difference among the groups). The most effective drug was diltiazem. Diltiazem was the most effective drug in young and old blacks. while captopril was the most effective in young whites and atenolol in old whites. The least effective drug in young and old blacks was captopril, while hydrochlorothiazide was the least effective in young whites and prazosin in old whites. Intolerance to medication during the titration phase was more common with clonidine and prazosin than the other drugs.

Conclusions

Among men, age and race are important determinants of the response to monotherapy for hypertension.

BBB

Behandla Blodtryck Bättre (Treat Blood Pressure Better)

Title	The BBB study: the effect of intensified antihypertensive treatment on the level of blood pressure, side-effects, morbidity and mortality in "well-treated" hypertensive patients.
Authors	Hansson L, for the BBB study group.
Reference	Blood Press 1994;3:248-254.
Disease	Hypertension.
Purpose	To investigate whether it is feasible to lower the diastolic blood pressure further through intensified therapy without an increase in side effects, and whether such intensified therapy will reduce morbidity and mortality.
Design	Randomized, open label, multicenter.
Patients	2127 patients, age 46-71 years, with essential hypertension (diastolic blood pressure 90-100 mmHg).
Follow-up	>4 years.
Treatment regimen	Intensified therapy (use of pharmacologic and non pharmacologic means to reduce diastolic blood pressure ≤80 mmHg) or unchanged therapy (maintain diastolic blood pressure 90-100 mmHg).
Additional therapy	No restriction on medications.

Results

With intensified therapy blood pressure fell from 155/95 to 141/83 mmHg (a difference of 14/12 mmHg, $p<0.001/0.001$). In the conventional therapy, blood pressure declined from 155/94 to 152/91 mmHg (a difference of 3/3 mmHg, $p<0.05/0.05$). A difference in diastolic blood pressure of 7-8.5 mmHg between the groups persisted for more than 4 years. In both groups there was no difference in heart rate between baseline and at the end of the study. Fewer adverse effects were reported in the intensified than conventional therapy group. There was no significant difference between the intensified and conventional therapy groups in the rates of stroke (8 vs 11 patients), myocardial infarction (20 vs 18 patients). No data on mortality was provided.

Conclusions

Blood pressure can be further reduced in intensified therapy without increment of adverse effects. However, it was not associated with improved outcome.

ACCT

Amlodipine Cardiovascular Community Trial

Title	Sex and age-related antihypertensive effects of amlodipine.
Authors	Kloner RA, Sowers JR, DiBona GF, et al.
Reference	Am J Cardiol 1996;77:713-722.
Disease	Hypertension.
Purpose	To assess whether there are age, sex, or racial differences in the response to amlodipine 5-10 mg/d in patients with mild to moderate hypertension.
Design	Open label, multicenter.
Patients	1084 patients, age 21-80 years, with mild to moderate hypertension (diastolic blood pressure 95-110 mmHg on 2 visits). Patients with history of stroke or transient ischemic attack, myocardial infarction within 6 months, angina pectoris, ventricular ejection fraction <40%, NYHA class ≥II heart failure, arrhythmias, or other systemic diseases were excluded.
Follow-up	18 weeks.
Treatment regimen	A 2-week placebo run-in phase, a 4-week titration/efficacy phase- amlodipine 5-10 mg/d was administered once daily, a 12-week maintenance phase, and an optional long-term follow-up phase.
Additional therapy	All other antihypertensive medications were not permitted.

ACCT

Amlodipine Cardiovascular Community Trial

(continued)

Results At the end of the titration/efficacy phase, mean decrease in blood pressure was 16.3±12.3/ 12.5±5.9 mmHg ($p<0.0001$). 86% of the patients achieved diastolic blood pressure ≤90 mmHg and/or a 10 mmHg decrease in diastolic blood pressure. The blood pressure response was greater in women (91.4%) than men (83.0%, $p<0.001$), and in those ≥65 years (91.5%) than those <65 years old (84.1%, $p<0.01$). 86.0% and 85.9% of the whites and blacks responded (p=NS). Amlodipine was well tolerated. Mild to moderate edema was the most common adverse effect. 14.6% discontinued therapy during the titration phase. Discontinuation due to adverse effects related to the drug occurred in 2.4%. During the maintenance phase 5.9% discontinued medication due to adverse effects (5.1% due to adverse effects possibly related to amlodipine).

Conclusions Amlodipine was effective and relatively safe as a once-a-day monotherapy for mild to moderate hypertension in a community-based population. The response rate in women was greater than in men.

Title	Evaluation of blood pressure response to the combination of enalapril (single dose) and diltiazem ER (four different doses) in systemic hypertension.
Authors	Applegate WB, Cohen JD, Wolfson P, et al.
Reference	Am J Cardiol 1996;78:51-55.
Disease	Hypertension.
Purpose	To assess the efficacy, safety, and dose-response of a combination of enalapril with a new once-daily formulation of diltiazem.
Design	Randomized, double blind, placebo controlled, multicenter.
Patients	336 patients, 21-75 years of age, with essential hypertension (diastolic blood pressure 95-115 mmHg). Patients with myocardial infarction within 2 years, secondary hypertension, previous cerebrovascular event, congestive heart failure, serious cardiac arrhythmias, or angina pectoris were excluded.
Follow-up	6 weeks.
Treatment regimen	After 7-day washout period, patients underwent 4-week single-blind placebo baseline phase. Then, patients entered the 6-week double blind treatment phase: randomization to one of six groups. 1. Placebo; 2. Enalapril 5 mg/d (E5); 3. Enalapril 5 mg/d and diltiazem ER 60 mg/d (E5/D60); 4. Enalapril 5 mg/d and diltiazem ER 120 mg/d (E5/D120); 5. Enalapril 5 mg/d and diltiazem ER 180 mg/d (E5/D180); 6. Enalapril 5 mg/d and diltiazem ER 240 mg/d (E5/D240).
Additional therapy	β blockers, digitalis, any medication that could lower blood pressure, psychotropic agents, and cimetidine were prohibited.

Results

By the end of the 6-week treatment period, diastolic blood pressure was reduced by 3.2 mmHg in the placebo; 5.6 mmHg in the E5; 6.8 mmHg in the E5/D60; 8.3 mmHg in the E5/D120; 10.1 mmHg in the E5/D180; and 10.3 mmHg in the E5/D240 group ($p<0.05$ for each group vs placebo). There was a significant linear dose-response relation ($p<0.001$). Diastolic blood pressure <90 mmHg was found in 25.5% of the E5/D60, 43.1% of the E5/D120, 40.0% of the E5/D180, and 49.1% of the E5/D240 groups. Only the enalapril alone (8.2 mmHg) and the three higher diltiazem doses (7.9, 12.8, and 13.8 mmHg in the E5/D120, E5/D180, and E5/D240 groups) resulted in a significant reduction of systolic blood pressure ($p<0.05$), whereas systolic blood pressure was reduced by only 2.0 and 6.5 mmHg in the placebo and E5/D60 groups, respectively. Drug related adverse effects were noted in 8.6% of the placebo group, 14.3% of the E5 group, and in 8.9% to 19.0% of the four combination groups.

Conclusions

A combination of low dose of enalapril and diltiazem ER was effective in lowering blood pressure in mild to moderately hypertensive patients. The combination of E5/D180 appeared to be the optimal dosage for reduction of blood pressure with acceptable rate of adverse events.

Title	Combined enalapril and felodipine extended release (ER) for systemic hypertension.
Authors	Gradman AH, Cutler NR, Davis PJ, et al.
Reference	Am J Cardiol 1997;79:431-435.
Disease	Hypertension.
Purpose	To assess the efficacy and safety of combination antihypertensive therapy with enalapril and felodipine extended release in patients with essential hypertension.
Design	Randomized, double blind, placebo controlled, multicenter, 3X4 factorial design.
Patients	707 patients, mean age 53.3 years, with essential hypertension (diastolic blood pressure 95-115 mmHg). Patients with creatinine clearance <60 ml/min, hepatic dysfunction, recent myocardial infarction, or congestive heart failure were excluded.
Follow-up	8 weeks.
Treatment regimen	4-week single-blind placebo baseline phase, thereafter randomization to placebo, enalapril (5 or 20 mg), felodipine ER (2.5, 5, or 10 mg), or their combinations for 8-weeks.

Results

All doses of felodipine and enalapril had a statistically significant ($p<0.05$) additive effect in reducing both diastolic and systolic blood pressures. The estimated reduction of diastolic blood pressure was 4.4 mmHg in the placebo, 6.0 mmHg in the enalapril 5 mg/d and 8.1 mmHg in the enalapril 20 mg/d, whereas the reduction in diastolic blood pressure was 7.3, 9.2, and 11.7 mmHg for the felodipine 2.5, 5, and 10 mg/d alone, respectively. The estimated reduction in diastolic blood pressure was 8.9, 10.8, and 13.3 mmHg for the combination of enalapril 5 mg/d with felodipine 2.5, 5, and 10 mg/d respectively, and 11.0, 12.9, and 15.4 mmHg for the combination of enalapril 20 mg/d with felodipine 2.5, 5, and 10 mg/d respectively. The estimated trough to peak ratio for sitting diastolic blood pressure ranged from 0.63 for enalapril 5 mg/d + felodipine 2.5 mg/d to 0.65 for enalapril 5 mg/d + felodipine 5 mg/d and 0.79 for enalapril 20 mg/d + felodipine 10 mg/d. The estimated percentage of patients with good or excellent blood pressure reduction ranged from 24.0% in the placebo group, 36.5% and 44.4% for the enalapril 5 and 20 mg/d alone, 39.6%, 54.0%, and 66.3% for the felodipine 2.5, 5, and 10 mg/d alone, to 52.1% for the combination of felodipine 2.5 mg/d and enalapril 5 mg/d and 86.7% for the combination of felodipine 10 mg/d and enalapril 20 mg/d. Patients ≥65 years old had greater reduction in diastolic blood pressure than younger patients. Combinations of felodipine and enalapril were associated with less drug-induced peripheral edema (4.1%) than felodipine alone (10.8%). Dizziness was reported in 4.4% of the combinations group vs 2.8% of the felodipine alone and 1.5% of the enalapril alone groups. There were no serious drug-related adverse effects.

Conclusions

Combination antihypertensive therapy with felodipine ER and enalapril was effective, safe, and well tolerated.

Low-Dose Reserpine-Thiazide Combination versus Nitrendipine Monotherapy

Title	Different concepts in first-line treatment of essential hypertension. Comparison of a low-dose reserpine-thiazide combination with nitrendipine monotherapy.
Authors	Krönig B, Pittrow DB, Kirch W, et al.
Reference	Hypertension 1997;29:651-658.
Disease	Hypertension.
Purpose	To compare the efficacy and tolerability of reserpine, clopamid, their combination, and nitrendipine.
Design	Randomized, double blind, parallel, multicenter.
Patients	273 patients, ≥18 years old, with essential hypertension (diastolic blood pressure 100-114 mmHg). Patients with drug or alcohol abuse, history of allergy, contraindications to one of the study medications, mental impairment, secondary hypertension, cerebrovascular event within 6 weeks, unstable angina or myocardial infarction within 3 months, severe heart failure or valvular heart disease, colitis, severe gastroenteritis, hepatic or renal impairment, depression, electrolyte disorders, and hyperlipidemia were excluded.
Follow-up	12 weeks.
Treatment regimen	4 week wash-out period followed by a 2 week single-blind placebo run-in phase and then, randomization to one of 4 groups: 1. Reserpine 0.1 to 0.2 mg/d; 2. Clopamid 5 to 10 mg/d; 3. Reserpine 0.1 mg/d + clopamid 5 mg/d; and 4. Nitrendipine 20 to 40 mg/d. If diastolic blood pressure remained ≥90 mmHg after 6 weeks, the medication dose was doubled.

Additional therapy

The use of digitalis and nitroglycerin was permitted. Nonsteroidal anti-inflammatory agents, steroids, psychotropic or antidepressant drugs were prohibited.

Results

Compliance was not less than 95.4% in all study groups at any visit. After 6 weeks of therapy with one capsule daily, mean reductions in sitting systolic/diastolic blood pressure from baseline was 14.0/11.7 mmHg in the reserpine, 13.6/11.9 mmHg in the clopamid, 11.6/12.3 mmHg in the nitrendipine, and 23.0/17.1 mmHg in the reserpine-clopamid combination group ($p<0.01$). 39.7% of the reserpine, 36.2% of the clopamid, 33.3% of the nitrendipine, and 55.2% of the combination therapy group achieved diastolic blood pressure <90 mmHg. Doubling of the respective medication dosage in the patients in whom diastolic blood pressure remained ≥90 mmHg after the 6th week resulted in normalization of diastolic blood pressure in 35.3% of the reserpine, 39.1% of the clopamid, 44.9% of the nitrendipine, and 65.7% of the combination therapy group ($p<0.0001$). Linear regression modeling indicated that the combination of reserpine and clopamid acted more than additively. 28% of the reserpine, 29% of the clopamid, 48% of the nitrendipine, and 27% of the combination therapy group had one or more adverse effects ($p<0.05$). Serious adverse effects were found in 0, 1%, 1%, and 0, respectively. Withdrawal from the study because of adverse effects occurred in 3%, 7%, 13%, and 3%, respectively ($p=0.06$). The percentage of patients whose diastolic blood pressure was normalized and remained free of any adverse event was 40% in the combination therapy group, 19% in the reserpine group, 20% in the clopamid group, and 12% in the nitrendipine group ($p<0.0001$).

Conclusions

A low-dose combination therapy with reserpine and clopamid was more effective than either drug alone or nitrendipine alone in lowering blood pressure. The combination therapy was well tolerated and safe. Reserpine, clopamid and nitrendipine as monotherapy were associated with relatively low success rates.

Title	Fosinopril verus enalapril in the treatment of hypertension: a double-blind study in 195 patients.
Authors	Hansson L, Forslund T, Höglund C, et al.
Reference	J Cardiovasc Pharmacol 1996;28:1-5.
Disease	Hypertension.
Purpose	To compare the efficacy of two angiotensin-converting-enzyme inhibitors, fosinopril and enalapril in reducing blood pressure in patients with essential hypertension.
Design	Randomized, double blind, multicenter.
Patients	195 patients, 18-80 years old, with mild to moderate essential hypertension (supine diastolic blood pressure 95-110 mmHg). Patients with collagen vascular disease, significant cardiac, renal, hepatic, hematologic, or cerebrovascular disease were excluded.
Follow-up	24 weeks.
Treatment regimen	After 4 weeks of placebo period, patients were randomized to fosinopril 20 to 40 mg/d or enalapril 10 to 20 mg/d. If supine diastolic blood pressure remained >90 mmHg, hydrochlorothiazide 12.5 mg was added.

Results

After 8 weeks of therapy diastolic blood pressure had decreased by 8.3 mmHg ($p<0.01$) in the fosinopril group and by 7.3 mmHg ($p<0.01$) in the enalapril group, whereas systolic blood pressures were reduced by 10.6 mmHg in both groups. After 8 weeks, the medication dose was doubled in 42% of the fosinopril group and 49% of the enalapril group. At week 16, hydrochlorothiazide was added to 27% of the fosinopril vs 30% of the enalapril-treated patients. By the end of the 24th week, there was no difference in reduction of either diastolic (10.7 vs 10.5 mmHg) or systolic blood pressure (14.7 vs 14.5 mmHg) between the fosinopril and enalapril groups. 8 patients in the fosinopril group vs 14 in the enalapril group were withdrawn from the study due to adverse effects. Adverse effects were reported in 58% and 67%, respectively. Serum angiotensin converting enzyme activity was significantly lower during fosinopril therapy than during enalapril therapy.

Conclusions

Fosinopril was equally effective as enalapril in reducing blood pressure in mild to moderate essential hypertension. Fosinopril was associated with better inhibition of the serum angiotensin-converting enzyme activity.

Title	Alpha-blockade and thiazide treatment of hypertension. A double-blind randomized trial comparing doxazosin and hydrochlorothiazide.
Authors	Grimm RH Jr, Flack JM, Schoenberger JA, et al.
Reference	Am J Hypertension 1996;9:445-454.
Disease	Hypertension.
Purpose	To compare the effect of hydrochlorothiazide and the $\alpha 1$ blocker doxazosin in patients with hypertension.
Design	Randomized, double-blind, parallel.
Patients	107 patients with hypertension.
Follow-up	1 year.
Treatment regimen	Hydrochlorothiazide (25 to 50 mg/d) or doxazosin (2 to 16 mg/d).

Results	Both drugs were well tolerated. Only 4% of the doxazosin and 7% of the hydrochlorothiazide-treated patients were withdrawn from the study. Both drugs were equally effective in controlling hypertension. After 1 year of treatment systolic/diastolic blood pressure was reduced, compared to baseline, by 19/16 mmHg in the doxazosin and by 22/15 in the hydrochlorothiazide groups. Sitting heart rate was not affected by the drugs. There was no evidence of tolerance development to either drug. Average final doses were 7.8 mg for doxazosin and 36 mg for hydrochlorothiazide. Changes in quality of life scores were comparable between the groups.
Conclusions	Over 1 year of therapy, both hydrochlorothiazide and doxazosin were effective in treating hypertension.

Losartan versus Placebo and Enalapril

Title	An in-patient trial of the safety and efficacy of losartan compared with placebo and enalapril in patients with essential hypertension.
Authors	Byyny RL, Merrill DD, Bradstreet TE, Sweet CS.
Reference	Cardiovasc Drugs Ther 1996;10:313-319.
Disease	Hypertension.
Purpose	To compare the effects of losartan, a specific and selective angiotensin II (subtype 1) receptor antagonist, and enalapril, an angiotensin converting enzyme inhibitor in patients with mild to moderate essential hypertension.
Design	Randomized, double blind, placebo-controlled multicenter.
Patients	100 in-patients, 21-72 years old (mean age 54 years), within 30% of their ideal body weight, with mild to moderate hypertension (supine diastolic blood pressure 95-120 mmHg). Black patients were not included. Patients with concomitant active medical problems that might have affected the antihypertensive therapy were excluded.
Follow-up	6 days.
Treatment regimen	After a 2 week outpatient single-blind placebo phase, patients were hospitalized for 2 days to determine patient eligibility for randomization, then a 5 day in-patient double-blind treatment phase, and a 1 day off-drug phase. Patients were randomized to placebo, losartan 50, 100, or 150 mg/d or enalapril 10 mg/d.
Additional therapy	ß blockers, digitalis, diuretics, angiotensin converting enzyme inhibitors, nitrates, and calcium channel blockers were prohibited.

Results

Diastolic and systolic blood pressure decreased in all five treatment groups, as compared with the placebo group ($p \leq 0.05$). The magnitude of the blood pressure response to 50 mg/d losartan was comparable at 24 hours to that achieved with enalapril 10 mg/d. There was an apparent plateauing of response with losartan, indicating no further decrease in mean diastolic blood pressure with doses >50 mg/d on the fifth day of therapy. The area under the 24 h blood pressure curve was comparable among the treatment groups on day 5. No rebound hypertension was observed after discontinuation of the study medications on day 6. Any adverse effects were noted in 48% of the placebo, 60% of the losartan 50 mg/d, 56% of the losartan 100 mg/d, 55% of the losartan 150 mg/d, and in 63% of the enalapril 10 mg/d group. Drug-related adverse effects were noted in 17%, 30%, 28%, 30%, and 42%, respectively. There were no serious clinical adverse effects.

Conclusions

Losartan was effective and safe in treating patients with mild to moderate essential hypertension.

6. Congestive Heart Failure

Title	Xamoterol in severe heart failure.
Authors	The Xamoterol in Severe Heart Failure Study Group.
Reference	Lancet 1990;336:1-6.
Disease	Congestive heart failure.
Purpose	To evaluate the efficacy and safety of xamoterol therapy for heart failure.
Design	Randomized, double blind, placebo controlled, multicenter.
Patients	516 patients, >18 years old, with NYHA class III and IV heart failure despite therapy with diuretics and an angiotensin converting enzyme inhibitor. Patients with myocardial infarction within 8 weeks, and premenopausal women were excluded.
Follow-up	Clinical evaluation and exercise test at baseline and after an average of 86 days for the placebo and 87 days for the xamoterol.
Treatment regimen	Xamoterol 200 mg X2/d or placebo.
Additional therapy	Any drug that influenced the ß adrenoreceptors was not permitted. Digitalis was allowed.

Results

There was no significant change in body weight at the end of the protocol for either group. Except for heart rate (79 vs 83 bpm, $p<0.01$) there was no difference in clinical signs between the groups. Visual analogue scale (11% vs 0%, $p<0.02$) and Likert scale (8% vs 2%, $p=0.02$) indicated that breathlessness improved with xamoterol. However, there was no difference in either the symptoms of fatigue, or exercise duration or total work done. Xamoterol did not affect the number of ventricular premature beats after exercise, and had no proarrhythmogenic activity. More patients in the xamoterol group withdrew from the study (19% vs 12%). On intention to treat analysis 9.2% of the xamoterol and 3.7% of the placebo died within 100 days (hazard ratio 2.54, 95% CI 1.04-6.18, $p=0.02$). Death due to progression of heart failure occurred in 1.2% and 4.8% of the placebo and xamoterol groups, while sudden death in 1.8% and 3.7%, respectively.

Conclusions

Xamoterol therapy resulted in excess of mortality, and was not associated with objective measures of improvement of exercise capacity. The study was terminated prematurely by the safety committee.

PROMISE

Prospective Randomized Milrinone Survival Evaluation Trial

Title	Effect of milrinone on mortality in severe chronic heart failure.
Authors	Packer M, Carver JR, Rodeheffer RJ, et al.
Reference	N Engl J Med 1991;325:1468-1475.
Disease	Congestive heart failure.
Purpose	To investigate the effects of milrinone on survival of patients with severe chronic heart failure.
Design	Randomized, double blind, placebo controlled, multicenter.
Patients	1088 patients with chronic heart failure NYHA class III-IV, with left ventricular ejection fraction ≤0.35. Patients who received ß blockers, calcium channel blockers, disopyramide, flecainide, encainide, dopamine or dobutamine were excluded.
Follow-up	1 day to 20 months (median 6.1 months).
Treatment regimen	Milrinone 10 mg X4/d or placebo PO.
Additional therapy	All patients received digoxin, diuretics, angiotensin converting enzyme inhibitors. Nitrates, hydralazine, prazosin, and other vasodilators were permitted.

PROMISE

Prospective Randomized Milrinone Survival Evaluation Trial

(continued)

Results

Mortality was 30% in the milrinone and 24% in the placebo group. Milrinone was associated with a 28% increase in total mortality (95% CI 1-61%, p=0.038), and with 34% increase in cardiovascular mortality (95% CI 6-69%, p=0.016). The adverse effect of milrinone was more pronounced in patients with NYHA class IV (53% increase in mortality, 95% CI 13-107%, p=0.006) than in patients with class III- 3% increase, 95% CI -28% to 48%, p=0.86). Milrinone did not have a beneficial effect on survival of any subgroup. Patients treated with milrinone had more hospitalization (44% vs 39%, p=0.041), and had more serious adverse cardiovascular reactions, including hypotension (11.4% vs 6.5% ,p=0.006) and syncope (8.0% vs 3.8%, p=0.002).

Conclusions

Long term therapy with milrinone increased the mortality and morbidity of patients with severe heart failure.

SOLVD- Treatment Study

Studies of Left Ventricular Dysfunction

Title	a. Studies of left ventricular dysfunction (SOLVD)- rationale, design and methods. Two trials that evaluate the effect of enalapril in patients with reduced ejection fraction. b. Effect of enalapril on survival in patients with reduced left ventricular ejection fractions and congestive heart failure.
Authors	The SOLVD Investigators.
Reference	a. Am J Cardiol 1990;66:315-322. b. N Engl J Med 1991;325:293-302.
Disease	Congestive heart failure, left ventricular dysfunction.
Purpose	To investigate whether enalapril therapy will reduce mortality and morbidity in patients with chronic heart failure and left ventricular ejection fraction ≤0.35.
Design	Randomized, double blind, placebo controlled, multicenter.
Patients	2569 Patients, age 21-80, with chronic heart failure and left ventricular ejection fraction ≤0.35. Patients with active angina pectoris requiring surgery, unstable angina, myocardial infarction within 1 month, renal failure or pulmonary disease were excluded. Patients already on angiotensin converting enzyme inhibitor therapy were excluded. Only patients that could tolerate enalapril 2.5 mg X2/d for 2-7 days were included.
Follow-up	22-55 months (average 41.4 months).
Treatment regimen	Enalapril (2.5 or 5mg X2/d initially, with gradual increase to 10 mg X2/d) or placebo.
Additional therapy	No restriction, except for other angiotensin converting enzyme inhibitors.

SOLVD- Treatment Study

Studies of Left Ventricular Dysfunction

(continued)

Results

39.7% of the placebo and 35.2% of the enalapril patients died (risk reduction 16%, 95% CI 5-26%, p=0.0036). Cardiovascular deaths occurred in 35.9% and 31.1%, respectively (risk reduction 18% (6-28%), p<0.002). The major difference was in death due to progressive heart failure (19.5% vs 16.3%, risk reduction 22% (6-35%), p=0.0045). 57.3% and 47.7% of the placebo and enalapril patients died or were hospitalized due to heart failure (risk reduction 26% (18-34%), p<0.0001). After 1 year there were 31.2% such events in the placebo and 20.4% in the enalapril (risk reduction 40% (30-48%)). 74% of the placebo and 69% of the enalapril patients were hospitalized at least once (p=0.006), 63% and 57% of the patients were hospitalized for primarily cardiovascular reasons (p<0.001).

Conclusions

Enalapril added to conventional therapy significantly reduced mortality and hospitalizations in patients with chronic heart failure due to systolic dysfunction.

V-HeFT II

Vasodilator Heart Failure Trial II

Title	A comparison of enalapril with hydralazine-isosorbide dinitrate in the treatment of chronic congestive heart failure.
Authors	Cohn JN, Johnson G, Zeische S, et al.
Reference	N Engl L Med 1991;325:303-310.
Disease	Congestive heart failure.
Purpose	To compare the effects of hydralazine-isosorbide dinitrate and enalapril in the treatment of congestive heart failure.
Design	Randomized, double blind, multicenter.
Patients	804 men, age 18-75 years, with chronic congestive heart failure (cardiothoracic ratio≥0.55 on chest radiography, LV internal diameter at diastole >2.7 cm/m^2 body surface area on echocardiography, or LVEF<0.45 on radionuclide scan) and reduced exercise tolerance. Patients with active angina were excluded.
Follow-up	0.5-5.7 years (mean 2.5 years).
Treatment regimen	1. Enalapril 10 mg X2/d. 2. Hydralazine 75 mg X4/d and isosorbide dinitrate 40 mg X4/d.
Additional therapy	Digoxin and diuretics

V-HeFT II

Vasodilator Heart Failure Trial II

(continued)

Results

2 year mortality was lower in the enalapril arm (18%) than the hydralazine arm (25%, p=0.016) which was attributed to a reduction of sudden death, especially in patients with NYHA class I or II. The reduction in mortality with enalapril was 33.6%, 28.2%, 14.0%, and 10.3% after 1-, 2-, 3-, and 4-years. Body oxygen consumption at peak exercise was increased after 13 weeks and after 6 months only in the hydralazine-isosorbide dinitrate group (p<0.05). However, after one year, oxygen consumption began to decline in both groups. Left ventricular ejection fraction increased more during the first 13 weeks in the hydralazine-isosorbide dinitrate group (0.033 vs. 0.021, p<0.03). However, after 3 years there was no difference between the groups. An increase in the incidence of cough and symptomatic hypotension was noted in the enalapril group, and of headache in the hydralazine-isosorbide dinitrate group.

Conclusions

While enalapril improved survival better than hydralazine-isosorbide dinitrate, the improvement of left ventricular ejection fraction and exercise capacity was greater with hydralazine-isosorbide dinitrate. A combination of these drugs may enhance their efficacy.

SOLVD- Prevention Study

Studies of Left Ventricular Dysfunction

Title	a. Studies of left ventricular dysfunction (SOLVD)- rationale, design and methods. Two trials that evaluate the effect of enalapril in patients with reduced ejection fraction. b. Effect of enalapril on mortality and the development of heart failure in asymptomatic patients with reduced left ventricular ejection fractions.
Authors	The SOLVD Investigators.
Reference	a. Am J Cardiol 1990;66:315-322. b. N Engl J Med 1992;327:685-691.
Disease	Congestive heart failure, left ventricular dysfunction.
Purpose	To investigate whether enalapril therapy will reduce mortality and morbidity in asymptomatic patients with left ventricular dysfunction.
Design	Randomized, double blind, placebo controlled, multicenter.
Patients	4228 patients, age 21-80, with left ventricular ejection fraction ≤ 0.35, who did not receive therapy for heart failure. However, diuretic therapy for hypertension and digoxin for atrial fibrillation were permitted.
Follow-up	Clinical follow-up for an average of 37.4 months (range 14.6-62.0 months).
Treatment regimen	Enalapril (2.5 mg X2/d initially, with gradual increase to 10 mg X2/d) or placebo.
Additional therapy	No restriction, except for other angiotensin converting enzyme inhibitors.

SOLVD- Prevention Study

Studies of Left Ventricular Dysfunction

(continued)

Results

Total mortality was 15.8% and 14.8% in the placebo and enalapril groups (reduction of risk 8%, 95% CI -8% to 21%, p=0.30). The difference was entirely due to a reduction in cardiovascular death (14.1% vs 12.6%, respectively, risk reduction 12%, 95% CI -3% to 26%, p=0.12). Heart failure developed in 30.2% vs 20.7% of the placebo and enalapril patients (risk reduction 37%, 95% CI 28% to 44%, p<0.001). The median length of time to development of heart failure was 8.3 vs 22.3 months, respectively. Hospitalization due to heart failure occurred in 12.9% vs 8.7%, respectively (p<0.001). The median length of time to the first hospitalization for heart failure was 13.2 vs 27.8 months, respectively.

Conclusions

Enalapril therapy delayed the development of heart failure and reduced the rate of related hospitalizations among patients with asymptomatic left ventricular dysfunction. There was also a trend toward decreased cardiovascular mortality in the enalapril group.

MDC

Metoprolol in Dilated Cardiomyopathy

Title	Beneficial effects of metoprolol in idiopathic dilated cardiomyopathy.
Authors	Waagstein F, Bristow MR, Swedberg K, et al.
Reference	Lancet 1993;342:1441-1446.
Disease	Congestive heart failure, dilated cardiomyopathy.
Purpose	To evaluate the effect of metoprolol therapy upon survival and morbidity in patients with dilated cardiomyopathy.
Design	Randomized, double blind, placebo controlled, multicenter.
Patients	383 patients, 16-75 years old, with dilated cardiomyopathy (ejection fraction <0.40). Patients treated with ß blockers, calcium channel blockers, inotropic drugs (except digoxin), or high doses of tricyclic antidepressant drugs were excluded. Patients with significant coronary artery disease, active myocarditis, chronic obstructive lung disease, insulin dependent diabetes, and alcoholism were not included. Only patients that could tolerate metoprolol 5 mg X2/d for 2-7 days were included.
Follow-up	Clinical follow-up for 12-18 months. Exercise test, right heart catheterization, and radionuclide ventriculography at baseline, 6 and 12 months.
Treatment regimen	Placebo or metoprolol. The target dose was 100-150 mg/d for 12-18 months.
Additional therapy	Digitalis, diuretics, angiotensin converting enzyme inhibitors and nitrates were permitted.

Metoprolol in Dilated Cardiomyopathy

(continued)

Results

The primary end point of death or need for cardiac transplantation was reached by 20.1% of the placebo and 12.9% of the metoprolol group (34% risk reduction, 95% CI -6 to 62%, p=0.058). 10.1% vs 1.0% of the placebo and metoprolol patients needed cardiac transplantation (p=0.0001). However, there was no difference in mortality alone (10.0% vs 11.9%, respectively). Mean ejection fraction was similar at baseline (0.22±0.09 vs 0.22±0.08). However, ejection fraction increased more in the metoprolol group after 6 months (0.26±0.11 vs 0.32±0.13 (p <0.0001)) and after 12 months (0.28±0.12 vs 0.34±0.14 (p<0.0001)). The improvement in ejection fraction was independent of the use of other medications and on the initial ejection fraction. Quality of life improved more in the metoprolol group (p=0.01). Exercise time at 12 months was significantly longer (p=0.046) in the metoprolol group. Heart rate and pulmonary wedge pressure decreased significantly more in the metoprolol than in the placebo group, whereas systolic pressure, stroke volume, and stroke work index increased more with metoprolol.

Conclusions

Metoprolol reduced clinical deterioration, improved symptoms and cardiac function and was well tolerated. However, mortality was not reduced.

FACET

Flosequinan-ACE Inhibitor Trial

Title	Can further benefit be achieved by adding flosequinan to patients with congestive heart failure who remain symptomatic on diuretic, digoxin, and an angiotensin converting enzyme inhibitor? Results of the Flosequinan-ACE Inhibitor Trial (FACET).
Authors	Massie BM, Berk MR, Brozena SC, et al.
Reference	Circulation 1993;88:492-501.
Disease	Congestive heart failure.
Purpose	To evaluate whether the addition of flosequinan to angiotensin converting enzyme inhibitors, diuretics and digoxin will improve exercise tolerance and quality of life of patients with congestive heart failure.
Design	Randomized, double blind, placebo controlled, multicenter.
Patients	322 patients, ≥18 years old, with congestive heart failure ≥12 weeks, left ventricular ejection fraction ≤35%, and were able to exercise to an end point of dyspnea or fatigue. All patients were on angiotensin converting enzyme inhibitor and diuretic therapy for ≥12 weeks.
Follow-up	Clinical follow-up, 24 h ECG monitoring, and repeated exercise test for 16 weeks.
Treatment regimen	Placebo, flosequinan 100 mg X1/d, or flosequinan 75 mg X2/d. If the heart rate increased by ≥15 bpm, the dose was reduced to 75 mg X1/d or 50 mg X2/d.

FACET

Flosequinan-ACE Inhibitor Trial

(continued)

Additional therapy

calcium channel blockers, β or α blockers, long acting nitrates, disopyramide or other class Ic antiarrhythmic agents, theophylline, bronchodilators, or other investigational drugs were not permitted.

Results

After 16 weeks, exercise time increased by 64 s in the 100 mg/d flosequinan group compared with only 5 s in the placebo group ($p<0.05$), whereas the higher dose did not reach statistical significant improvement. Flosequinan 100 mg/d resulted in improvement of the Minnesota Living With Heart Failure Questionnaire (LWHF) score compared with placebo. Both flosequinan doses were associated with improvement of the physical score, whereas the 75 mg X2/d was associated with worsening of the emotional component. NYHA class was improved in 22.0% and worsened in 14.7% of the placebo group, while the corresponding rates for flosequinan 100 mg/d were 30.9% and 16.4%, and for flosequinan 75 mg X2/d 39.3% and 15.7%, respectively. There was no significant difference in mortality, hospitalization for all causes, hospitalization for heart failure, or withdrawal for worsening of heart failure among the groups. There was no increase in ventricular arrhythmias with flosequinan.

Conclusions

Flosequinan resulted in symptomatic benefit when added to angiotensin converting enzyme inhibitor and diuretic therapy for heart failure. However, in another study, the same dose resulted in an adverse effect on survival.

REFLECT

Randomized Evaluation of Flosequinan on Exercise Tolerance

Title	Double-blind, placebo-controlled study of the efficacy of flosequinan in patients with chronic heart failure.
Authors	Packer M, Narahara KA, Elkayam U, et al.
Reference	J Am Coll Cardiol 1993;22:65-72.
Disease	Congestive heart failure.
Purpose	To evaluate the effects of flosequinan on symptoms and exercise capacity in patients with chronic heart failure who remained symptomatic despite therapy with digitalis and diuretics.
Design	Randomized, double blind, placebo controlled, multicenter.
Patients	193 patients, ≥18 years old, with dyspnea or fatigue on exertion (NYHA II or III), left ventricular ejection fraction ≤40% and cardiothoracic ratio ≥50%. All patients were symptomatic despite therapy with digitalis and diuretics for ≥2 months. Patients with hypotension, angina, pulmonary renal or hepatic disease, claudication, or myocardial infarction within 3 months were excluded.
Follow-up	12 weeks of clinical follow-up and repeated exercise test and radionuclide ventriculography.
Treatment regimen	Flosequinan 100 mg/d or placebo in addition to diuretic agent and digoxin. If the dose was not tolerated, a dose of 75 mg/d was permitted.
Additional therapy	Use of other vasodilators was not permitted. Use of antiarrhythmic agents, except ß blockers, was permitted.

REFLECT

Randomized Evaluation of Flosequinan on Exercise Tolerance

(continued)

Results

After 12 weeks, maximal exercise time increased by 96 s in the flosequinan vs 47 s in the placebo group ($p=0.22$). Maximal oxygen consumption increased by 1.7 vs 0.6 ml/kg/min, respectively ($p=0.05$). By 12 weeks, 55% of the flosequinan vs 36% of the placebo treated patients improved their heart failure symptoms ($p=0.018$), while 10% vs 19% had worsening heart failure ($p=0.07$). Flosequinan did not change the functional class, cardiothoracic ratio, or ejection fraction. Seven vs 2 deaths occurred in the flosequinan and placebo groups, respectively ($p>0.10$).

Conclusions

Flosequinan therapy resulted in symptomatic improvement and an increase in exercise time. However, the effect on survival remains to be determined.

GESICA

Grupo de Estudio de la Sobrevida en la Insuficiencia Cardiaca en Argentina

Title	Randomized trial of low-dose amiodarone in severe congestive heart failure.
Authors	Doval HC, Nul DR, Grancelli HO, et al.
Reference	Lancet 1994;344:493-498.
Disease	Congestive heart failure, arrhythmia.
Purpose	To evaluate the effect of low dose amiodarone on survival of patients with severe heart failure.
Design	Randomized, multicenter.
Patients	516 patients with severe heart failure NYHA class II-IV with evidence of cardiac enlargement or reduced ejection fraction ≤ 0.35. Patients with thyroid dysfunction, concomitant serious disease, valvular heart disease, hypertrophic or restrictive cardiomyopathy, angina pectoris, history of sustained ventricular arrhythmias were excluded.
Follow-up	2 years.
Treatment regimen	Amiodarone 600 mg/d for 14 d, and then 300 mg/d for 2 years.
Additional therapy	Low sodium diet, diuretics, digitalis, and vasodilators. Antiarrhythmic agents were not permitted.

GESICA

Grupo de Estudio de la Sobrevida en la Insuficiencia Cardiaca en Argentina

(continued)

Results

Mortality was 41.4% in the control and 33.5% in the amiodarone group (risk reduction 28%, 95% CI 4-45%, p=0.024). Both sudden death and death due to progressive heart failure were reduced. Fewer patients in the amiodarone group died or were hospitalized due to worsening of heart failure (45.8% vs 58.2%, RR 31%, 95% CI 13-46%, p=0.0024). The beneficial effect was evident in all subgroups examined and was independent of the presence of nonsustained ventricular tachycardia. Side effects were reported in 6.1% of the amiodarone group and lead to drug withdrawal in 4.6%.

Conclusions

Low-dose amiodarone is a safe and effective treatment for reduction of mortality and morbidity in patients with severe heart failure.

CIBIS

The Cardiac Insufficiency Bisoprolol Study

Title	A randomizea trial of ß blockade in heart failure. The Cardiac Insufficiency Bisoprolol Study (CIBIS).
Authors	CIBIS Investigators and Committees.
Reference	Circulation 1994;90:1765-1773.
Disease	Congestive heart failure.
Purpose	To assess the effects of bisoprolol therapy on mortality in patients with heart failure.
Design	Randomized, double blind, placebo controlled, multicenter.
Patients	641 patients, 18-75 years of age, with chronic heart failure (NYHA class III or IV) treated with diuretics and vasodilators, and left ventricular ejection fraction <40%. Patients with heart failure due to hypertrophic or restrictive cardiomyopathy, or due to mitral or aortic valve disease, or within 3 months of myocardial infarction were excluded. Patients awaiting for coronary artery bypass grafting or cardiac transplantation were not included.
Follow-up	Mean follow-up 1.9±0.1 years.
Treatment regimen	Placebo or bisoprolol. Initial dose was 1.25 mg/d with gradual increase to 5 mg/d.
Additional therapy	diuretics and a vasodilator therapy. Digitalis and amiodarone were permitted. ß blockers or mimetic agents and phosphodiesterase inhibitors were prohibited. Only calcium channel blockers of the dihydropyridine type were allowed.

CIBIS

The Cardiac Insufficiency Bisoprolol Study

(continued)

Results

Bisoprolol was well tolerated. Premature withdrawal from treatment occurred in 25.5% of the placebo and 23.4% of the bisoprolol group (p=NS). Bisoprolol did not significantly reduce mortality (20.9% vs 16.6% in the placebo and bisoprolol group, RR 0.80, 95% CI 0.56-1.15, p=0.22). No significant difference was found in sudden death rate (5.3% vs 4.7%, respectively), or death due to documented ventricular tachycardia or fibrillation (2.2% vs 1.3%). However bisoprolol improved the functional status of the patients. Hospitalization for cardiac decompensation occurred in 28.0% vs 19.1% (p<0.01), and improvement by >1 NYHA class was noted in 15.0% vs 21.3%, respectively (p<0.03).

Conclusions

ß blockers conferred functional improvement in patients with severe heart failure. However, there was no improvement in survival.

Flosequinan vs Captopril in Chronic Heart Failure

Title	Long-term evaluation of treatment for chronic heart failure: a 1 year comparative trial of flosequinan and captopril.
Authors	Cowley AJ, McEntegart DJ, Hampton JR, et al.
Reference	Cardiovasc Drugs Ther 1994;8:829-836.
Disease	Congestive heart failure.
Purpose	To compare the efficacy of flosequinan and captopril in patients with moderate to severe heart failure who remained symptomatic despite optimal diuretic therapy.
Design	Randomized, double blind, multicenter.
Patients	209 patients with moderate to severe heart failure (NYHA class III-IV) despite ≥80 mg frusemide/d or an equivalent diuretic, and a cardiothoracic ratio >50% on a standard chest x-ray. Patients treated with vasodilators were excluded.
Follow-up	12 months of clinical follow-up and either repeated exercise test or corridor walk test.
Treatment regimen	Flosequinan (50 mg/d for 2 weeks and then 100 mg/d for 2 weeks and 150 mg/d thereafter) or captopril 12.5 mg X3/d for 2 weeks, 25 mg X3/d for additional 2 weeks and then, 50 mg X3/d.
Additional therapy	Other vasodilators were not permitted.

Results	64% of the flosequinan vs 40% of the captopril groups failed to complete the study due to death or withdrawal ($p<0.001$). There was no statistically significant difference in mortality (18.6% in the flosequinan vs 14.0% in the captopril groups, 38% increase risk of death with flosequinan, 95% CI -30% to 172%, p=0.29). Worsening of heart failure occurred in 12.7% vs 10.3%, respectively. There were more adverse effects in the flosequinan treated patients. Both medications had similar effects on treadmill exercise test. The mean increase in exercise time at 52 weeks was 117 vs 156 seconds in the flosequinan and captopril groups (p=0.57). The increase in corridor walk distance was 40 vs 62 meters, respectively (p=0.015).
Conclusions	Flosequinan had comparable long term efficacy to captopril. However, it is associated with a higher incidence of adverse events.

Carvedilol in Congestive Heart Failure Due to Ischemic Heart Disease

Title	a) Effects of Carvedilol, a vasodilator-ß blocker, in patients with congestive heart failure due to ischemic heart disease. b) Randomized, placebo-controlled trial of carvedilol in patients with congestive heart failure due to ischaemic heart disease.
Authors	a) Australia-New Zealand Heart Failure Research Collaborative Group. b) Australia/New Zealand Heart Failure Research Collaborative Group.
Reference	Circulation 1995;92:212-218. Lancet 1997;349:375-380.
Disease	Congestive heart failure.
Purpose	To evaluate the effects of carvedilol on symptoms, exercise performance and left ventricular function in patients with heart failure due to coronary artery disease.
Design	Randomized, double blind, placebo controlled, multicenter.
Patients	415 patients, with chronic stable heart failure NYHA class II or III due to ischemic heart disease, left ventricular ejection fraction of <45%. Patients with systolic blood pressure <90 mmHg, heart rate of <50 /min, heart block, coronary event or procedure within 4 weeks, primary myocardial or valvular disease, insulin dependent diabetes, chronic obstructive airway disease, renal impairment, current therapy with verapamil, β blockers or agonists were excluded.
Follow-up	a) Clinical follow-up for 6 months and repeated exercise test, radionuclide ventriculography and echocardiography at 6 months have been reported. b) Left ventricular radionuclide ventriculography, echocardiography, treadmill exercise duration, and clinical follow-up at baseline, 6 and 12 months. Average follow-up of 19 months.
Treatment regimen	2-3 weeks of open label carvedilol, started at 3.125 mgX2/d and increased to 6.25 mgX2/d. Patients who could tolerate the dose were randomized to placebo or carvedilol with gradual increments of the dose towards 25 mgX2/d
Additional therapy	Patients were treated with conventional therapy including angiotensin converting enzyme inhibitors, diuretics and digoxin.
Results	a). A total of 30 patients in the carvedilol vs 13 in the placebo group withdrew from the study (p=0.01), but no single cause accounted for the difference. After 6 months, left ventricular ejection fraction increased by 5.2% in the carvedilol group compared with placebo (95% CI 3.7%-6.8%, p<0.0001). Left ventricular end diastolic diameter did not change from baseline to 6 months of follow-up in the placebo group (68.1 vs 68.3 mm, respectively), whereas it decreased in the carvedilol

group (69.5 mm at baseline vs 68.3 mm at 6 months, p=0.048 for the difference between the groups). Left ventricular end systolic diameter did not change in the placebo group (56.1 vs 56.1 mm, respectively) whereas it decreased in the carvedilol group (57.3 mm at baseline vs 55.0 mm at follow-up, p=0.0005 for the difference between the groups). There was no change in exercise time between the groups after 6 months (mean difference -22 seconds, 95% CI -59 to 15 seconds). There was no difference in 6 min walk distance between the groups (mean difference -6 meter, 95% CI -18 to 6 meter). The severity of symptoms was unchanged in 67% of the of the placebo vs 65% of the carvedilol-treated patients. However, 28% of the placebo vs 23% of the carvedilol patients were improved according to NYHA classification, while 5% vs 12% were worsened (p=0.05). The same trend was present using the Specific Activity Scale (p=0.02). b) By the end of the follow-up, the numbers of withdrawals from the two groups were comparable (41 vs 30 in the carvedilol and placebo groups, respectively, p>0.1). After 12 months, left ventricular ejection fraction increased from 28.4% at baseline to 33.5% among the carvedilol assigned patients, whereas left ventricular ejection fraction did not change much in the placebo treated group. Therefore, at 12 months, left ventricular ejection fraction was 5.3% higher in the carvedilol than placebo group (p<0.0001). After 12 months, left ventricular end-diastolic and end-systolic dimensions were 1.7 mm (p=0.06) and 3.2 mm (p=0.001) smaller in the carvedilol compared with the placebo group. There was no clear differences between the groups in 6 min walk distance, treadmill exercise duration, NYHA class, or Specific Activity Scale. After 19 months, there was no difference between the groups in the incidence of worsening of heart failure (82 vs 75 of the carvedilol and placebo groups ; relative risk 1.12; 95% CI 0.82-1.53) and mortality (20 vs 26, respectively; relative risk 0.76; 95% CI 0.42-1.36; p>0.1). However, the rate of death or hospitalization was lower in the carvedilol group (104 vs 131; relative risk 0.74; 95% CI 0.57-0.95; p=0.02).

Conclusions

a) In patients with heart failure due to coronary artery disease, 6 month therapy with carvedilol improved left ventricular function, but symptoms were slightly worsened. b) Twelve months of carvedilol therapy resulted in improvement in left ventricular ejection fraction and in decrease in end-systolic and end-diastolic dimensions. There was an overall reduction in the combined end-point of death or hospitalization. However, there was no effect on mortality, exercise performance, symptoms, or episodes of worsening of heart failure.

Amiodarone in Patients with Congestive Heart Failure and Asymptomatic Ventricular Arrhythmia.

Title	a. Amiodarone in patients with congestive heart failure and asymptomatic ventricular arrhythmia. b. Effect of amiodarone on clinical status and left ventricular function in patients with congestive heart failure.
Authors	a. Singh SN, Fletcher RD, Fisher SG, et al. b. Massie BM, Fisher SG, Deedwania PC, et al.
Reference	a. N Engl J Med 1995;333:77-82. b. Circulation 1996;93:2128-2134.
Disease	Congestive heart failure, arrhythmia.
Purpose	To evaluate the efficacy of amiodarone to reduce mortality in patients with heart failure and asymptomatic ventricular arrhythmias.
Design	Randomized, double blind, placebo-controlled, multicenter
Patients	674 patients with congestive heart failure, left ventricular ejection fraction of ≤0.40, and ≥10 PVCs/h, unaccompanied by symptoms.
Follow-up	Clinical follow-up and repeated 24 h ambulatory ECG monitoring for >1 year (median follow-up 45 months, range 0-54 months).
Treatment regimen	Placebo or amiodarone 800 mg/d for 14 days, then 400 mg/d for 50 weeks, and then 300 mg/d until the end of the study.
Additional therapy	All patients received vasodilator therapy. Digoxin and diuretics were permitted.

Amiodarone in Patients with Congestive Heart Failure and Asymptomatic Ventricular Arrhythmia.

(continued)

Results

During follow-up 39% of the amiodarone vs 42% of the placebo patients died (p=NS). The overall actuarial survival at 2 years was 69.4% vs 70.8%, respectively (p=0.6). At 2 years the rate of sudden death was 15% vs 19% in amiodarone and placebo (p=0.43). Amiodarone had no effect on mortality among patients with ischemic heart disease However, there was a trend toward less mortality with amiodarone therapy among the 193 patients with nonischemic heart disease (p=0.07). Survival without cardiac death or hospitalization for heart failure was significantly reduced in amiodarone treated patients with non-ischemic heart disease (relative risk 0.56 (95% CI 0.36-0.87); p=0.01), but not in patients with ischemic heart disease (relative risk 0.95 (0.73-1.24); p=0.69). Amiodarone was effective in suppressing ventricular arrhythmias. While left ventricular ejection fraction was comparable at baseline (24.9±8.3% in the amiodarone vs 25.7±8.2% in the placebo), ejection fraction was significantly improved in the amiodarone group (at 24 months 35.4±11.5% vs 29.8±12.2, p<0.001). However, this increase in ejection fraction was not associated with greater clinical improvement, less diuretic requirements, or fewer hospitalization for heart failure.

Conclusions

Although amiodarone therapy suppressed ventricular tachyarrhythmias and improved left ventricular function, it was not associated with improved outcome, except for reduction of cardiac mortality and hospitalization for heart failure among patients with non-ischemic cardiomyopathy.

MEXIS

Metoprolol and Xamoterol Infarction Study

Title a. Effects of ß receptor antagonists in patients with clinical evidence of heart failure after myocardial infarction: double blind comparison of metoprolol and xamoterol.
b. Effects of beta receptor antagonists on left ventricular function in patients with clinical evidence of heart failure after myocardial infarction. A double-blind comparison of metoprolol and xamoterol. Echocardiographic results from the metoprolol and xamoterol infarction study (MEXIS).

Authors a. Persson H, Rythe'n-Alder E, Melcher A, Erhardt L
b. Persson H, Eriksson SV, Erhardt L.

Reference a. Br Heart J 1995;74:140-148.
b. Eur Heart J 1996;17:741-749.

Disease Congestive heart failure.

Purpose To compare the effects of xamoterol and metoprolol on exercise time in patients with mild to moderate heart failure after myocardial infarction.

Design Randomized, double blind, single center.

Patients 210 patients, age 40-80 years, with evidence of heart failure at any time during the 5-7 days after myocardial infarction. Patients with NYHA class IV, hypertrophic cardiomyopathy, aortic stenosis, pulmonary disease or unstable angina were excluded.

Follow-up 12 months of clinical follow-up and repeated exercise test and echocardiography.

Treatment regimen Metoprolol 50 mgX2/d or xamoterol 100 mgX2/d for 1 day, and then the dose was doubled. The lowest dose allowed was 50 mg/d metoprolol and 100 mg/d xamoterol

---

MEXIS

Metoprolol and Xamoterol Infarction Study

(continued)

Additional therapy

Diuretics, digitalis, nitrates, and angiotensin converting enzyme inhibitors were allowed. Calcium channel blockers were not permitted.

Results

a. Exercise time increased at 3 months by 22% in the metoprolol and 29% in the xamoterol groups (p=NS). Improvements in quality of life, clinical signs of heart failure, and NYHA class were seen in both groups over 1 year. Breathlessness improved only with xamoterol (p=0.003 and p=0.046 vs metoprolol after 3 and 6 months, however, there was no difference at 12 months). 18 vs 22 patients of the metoprolol and xamoterol groups withdrew from the study during 1 year. 5 and 6 patients of the metoprolol and xamoterol patients died.

b. In the xamoterol-treated patients, there was an increase in E-point septal separation from 12.2 mm at baseline to 13.2 mm after 12 months, whereas in the metoprolol group it decreased from 12.4 mm to 11.1 mm (p<0.005). Fractional shortening decreased in the xamoterol group (from 26.0% to 25.0%) and increased in the metoprolol group (from 25.8% to 26.9%) (p<0.05). There were no significant differences between the groups concerning left ventricular end systolic and end diastolic dimensions.

Conclusions

a. The efficacy of xamoterol and metoprolol in improving exercise tolerance, quality of life, and signs of heart failure were comparable.

b. In contrast to metoprolol, xamoterol therapy was associated with impairment of left ventricualr systolic function in patients with heart failure after myocardial infarction.

Carvedilol Heart Failure Study

Title	The effect of carvedilol on morbidity and mortality in patients with chronic heart failure.
Authors	Packer M, Bristow MR, Cohn JN, et al.
Reference	N Engl J Med 1996;334:1349-1355.
Disease	Congestive heart failure.
Purpose	To evaluate the effects of carvedilol, a nonselective ß-blocker that also blocks α1-receptors and has antioxidant properties, on survival and hospitalization of patients with chronic heart failure.
Design	Randomized, double blind, placebo-controlled, multicenter.
Patients	1094 patients with symptomatic heart failure for ≥3 months and left ventricular ejection fraction ≤0.35, despite ≥2 months of treatment with diuretics and an angiotensin converting enzyme inhibitor. Patients with primary valvular heart disease, active myocarditis, ventricular tachycardia or advanced heart block not controlled by antiarrhythmic intervention or a pacemaker were excluded. Patients with systolic blood pressure >160 or <85 mmHg, heart rate <68 bpm, major cardiovascular event or surgery within 3 months, comorbidity that could affect survival or limit exercise capacity, or patients treated with ß blocker, calcium channel antagonist or class IC or III antiarrhythmics were not included.
Follow-up	6 months (12 months for the group with mild heart failure).
Treatment regimen	During the open-label phase, all patients received carvedilol 6.25 mgX2/d for 2 weeks. Patients who tolerated the drug were randomized on the basis of their baseline exercise capacity to one of 4 treatment protocols. Within each of the 4 protocols patients with mild, moderate, or severe heart failure were randomized to either carvedilol 12.5-50 mgX2/d or placebo.

Additional therapy Treatment with digoxin, hydralazine, or nitrate were permitted.

Results Of the 1197 patients that had entered the open-label phase, 5.6% failed to complete the period due to adverse effects. Another 3.0% violated the protocol. 1094 patients were randomized to the double-blind stage. The overall mortality was 7.8% in the placebo and 3.2% in the carvedilol group (65% reduction of risk, 95% CI 39-80%; $p<0.001$). Death from progressive heart failure was 3.3% in the placebo vs 0.7% in the carvedilol group. Sudden death occurred in 3.8% vs 1.7% of the placebo and carvedilol groups. The reduction in mortality was similar regardless of age, sex. the cause of heart failure, ejection fraction, exercise tolerance, systolic blood pressure, or heart rate. During the follow-up 19.6% vs 14.1% of the placebo and carvedilol groups were hospitalized at least once for cardiovascular causes (27% reduction of risk, 95% CI 3-45%; $p=0.036$). The combined end-point of hospitalization for cardiovascular causes or death was reduced by 38% (24.6% vs 15.8% in the placebo and carvedilol group; 95% CI 18-53%, $p<0.001$).

Conclusions Carvedilol reduces the risk of death and the risk of hospitalization for cardiovascular causes in patients with heart failure who are receiving treatment with digoxin, diuretics, and angiotensin converting enzyme inhibitor.

MOCHA

Multicenter Oral Carvedilol Heart failure Assessment

Title	Carvedilol produces dose-related improvements in left ventricular function and survival in subjects with chronic heart failure.
Authors	Bristow MR, Gilbert EM, Abraham WT, et al.
Reference	Circulation 1996;94:2807-2816.
Disease	Congestive heart failure.
Purpose	To assess the dose-response characteristics of carvedilol in patients with chronic heart failure.
Design	Randomized, double blind, placebo controlled, dose response evaluation, multicenter.
Patients	345 patients, aged 18 to 85 years, with left ventricular ejection fraction ≤0.35 and symptoms of stable heart failure for ≥3 months. All patients had to be treated with diuretics and angiotensin converting enzyme inhibitor for ≥1 month before entry. Patients had to be able to walk 150 to 450 m on the 6-min walk test. Patients with heart rate <68 bpm, uncorrected valvular disease, hypertrophic cardiomyopathy, uncontrolled ventricular tachycardia, sick sinus syndrome, advanced AV block, symptomatic peripheral vascular disease, severe concomitant disease, a stroke or myocardial infarction within 3 months, hypertension or hypotension were excluded. A PTCA, CABG or transplantation could not be planned or be likely for the 6 months after entry. Only patients that completed a 2 to 4-week challenge phase of open-label carvedilol 6.25 mgX2/d were included.
Follow-up	6 months.
Treatment regimen	Randomization to: 1. Placebo; 2. Carvedilol 6.25 mgX2/d; 3. Carvedilol 12.5 mgX2/d; or 4. Carvedilol 25 mgX2/d.

MOCHA

Multicenter Oral Carvedilol Heart failure Assessment

(continued)

Additional therapy

Diuretic therapy was mandatory. Angiotensin converting enzyme inhibitors were recommended. Digoxin, hydralazine and nitrates were permitted, if they had been started ≥2 months before entry. Calcium channel blockers, flosequinan, α or β blockers, anti-arrhythmic agents and monoamine oxidase inhibitors were not permitted.

Results

92% of subjects tolerated the open-label challenge period. Carvedilol therapy was not associated with an improvement in either the 6-minute corridor walk test or the 9-minute self-powered treadmill test. Similarly, there was no difference in the Minnesota Living With Heart Failure Questionnaire scores among the groups. However, carvedilol therapy resulted in a dose-related increase in left ventricular ejection fraction (by 5, 6, and 8% ejection fraction units in the low, medium and high dose carvedilol, compared with only 2 units in the placebo group; $p<0.001$ for the linear dose response). Carvedilol improved ejection fraction both in patients with ischemic and with non-ischemic cardiomyopathy. Carvedilol therapy was associated with lower cardiovascular hospitalization rate (mean number of hospitalization per patient 0.36, 0.14, 0.15, and 0.13, for the placebo, lower, medium and high carvedilol dose, respectively; $p=0.003$ for linear trend). Moreover, carvedilol reduced mortality (from 15.5% in the placebo group to 6.0% ($p<0.05$) , 6.7% ($p=0.07$), and 1.1% ($p<0.001$) in the low, medium and high carvedilol dose; $p<0.001$ for the linear trend). The reduction in mortality occurred both in patients with ischemic and non-ischemic cardiomyopathy. When the 3 carvedilol groups were combined, mortality risk was 73% lower than in the placebo group (relative risk 0.272; 95% CI 0.124 to 0.597; $p<0.001$).

Conclusions

In subjects with mild to moderate heart failure due to systolic dysfunction and who can tolerate carvedilol therapy, carvedilol treatment resulted in dose-related improvement in LV function and reduction in mortality and hospitalization rates.

Title	Carvedilol inhibits clinical progression in patients with mild symptoms of heart failure.
Authors	Colucci WS, Packer M, Bristow MR, et al.
Reference	Circulation 1996;94:2800-2806.
Disease	Congestive heart failure.
Purpose	To evaluate the effect of carvedilol in patients with mildly symptomatic heart failure.
Design	Randomized, double blind, placebo controlled, dose response evaluation, multicenter.
Patients	366 patients, 18-85 years old, with chronic stable symptomatic heart failure despite treatment with diuretics and an angiotensin converting enzyme inhibitor, and left ventricular ejection fraction $\leq$0.35. Patients with primary valvular disease; hypertrophic cardiomyopathy; symptomatic ventricular arrhythmias; myocardial infarction, unstable angina or CABG within 3 months; likelihood for revascularization or transplantation within 12 months; sick sinus syndrome or high degree AV block; hypotension or hypertension; or serious concomitant disease were excluded. Only patients who were able to walk 450 to 550 m on a 6-min walk test and tolerated a carvedilol 6.25 mgX2/d during a 2-week challenge open label phase were included in this protocol.
Follow-up	12 months of maintenance phase.
Treatment regimen	Randomization in a 2:1 ratio to carvedilol (n=232) or placebo (n=134). There was an initial 2 to 6 week double blind up-titration phase, beginning at 12.5 mgX2/d (maximum 25 mgX2/d for patients <85 kg; 50 mgX2/d for heavier patients).

Additional therapy

Diuretics and an angiotesnin converting enzyme inhibitor. Digoxin, hydralazine and nitrates were allowed. Antiarrhythmic drugs, calcium channel blockers, α or ß blockers, flosequinan and monoamine oxidase inhibitors were prohibited.

Results

Clinical progression of heart failure (defined as death due to heart failure, hospitalization for heart failure, or the need for a sustained increase in heart failure medications) occurred in 21% of the placebo group and in 11% of the carvedilol group (relative risk 0.52; 95% CI 0.32 to 0.85; p=0.008). This favorable effect was not influenced by gender, age, race, etiology of heart failure, or baseline left ventricular ejection fraction. 4.0% vs 0.9% of the placebo and carvedilol treated patients died (risk ratio 0.231; 95% CI 0.045 to 1.174; p=0.048). NYHA functional class improved in 12% of the carvedilol-treated patients vs 9% of the placebo-treated patients, whereas it worsened in 4% vs 15%, respectively (p=0.003). During the study more carvedilol than placebo treated patients stated that their symptoms improved (75% vs 60%; p=0.013). Similarly, the physician global assessment rated improvement in 69% vs 47% of the patients, respectively (p=0.001). However, there was no difference in the quality of life scores and the distance walked in 9-min treadmill test between the groups. At follow-up, the mean increase in left ventricular ejection fraction was larger in the carvedilol (0.10) than in the placebo (0.03) patients (p<0.001). The drug was well tolerated.

Conclusions

In patients with mildly symptomatic stable heart failure due to systolic dysfunction and who could tolerate carvedilol treatment, carvedilol reduced clinical progression of heart failure and mortality.

PRECISE

Prospective Randomized Evaluation of Carvedilol on Symptoms and Exercise

Title	Double-blind, placebo-controlled study of the effects of carvedilol in patients with moderate to severe heart failure. The Precise Trial.
Authors	Packer M, Colucci WS, Sackner-Bernstein JD, et al.
Reference	Circulation 1996;94:2793-2799.
Disease	Congestive heart failure.
Purpose	To evaluate the effect of carvedilol in patients with moderate to severe heart failure.
Design	Randomized, double blind, placebo controlled, dose response evaluation, multicenter.
Patients	278 patients, with chronic stable symptomatic heart failure despite treatment with diuretics and an angiotensin converting enzyme inhibitor for ≥2 months, and left ventricular ejection fraction ≤0.35. Patients with primary valvular disease; active myocarditis; restrictive or hypertrophic cardiomyopathy; symptomatic ventricular arrhythmias; myocardial infarction, unstable angina or CABG within 3 months; angina that limits exercise capacity; sick sinus syndrome or high degree AV block; hypotension or hypertension; stroke; peripheral vascular or pulmonary disease; or serious concomitant disease were excluded. Patients receiving antiarrhythmic drugs, calcium channel blockers, or α or ß blockers or agonists, were not included. Only patients who were able to walk 150 to 450 m on a 6-min walk test and tolerated carvedilol 6.25 mgX2/d during a 2-week challenge open label phase were included in this protocol.
Follow-up	Maintenance phase of 6 months.

PRECISE

Prospective Randomized Evaluation of Carvedilol on Symptoms and Exercise

(continued)

Treatment regimen

Randomization to placebo or carvedilol 12.5 mgX2/d. The dose was increased gradually to 25 mgX2/d (50 mgX2/d for patients >85 kg)

Additional therapy

Diuretics and an angiotensin converting enzyme inhibitor. Digoxin, hydralazine and nitrates were allowed. Antiarrhythmic drugs, calcium channel blockers, α or ßblockers or agonists were prohibited.

Results

Of the 301 patients entering the open-label phase, 23 (8%) did not complete it (17 patients due to adverse effects). By intention-to-treat analysis, the 6-min walk distance increased by 9 meter in the carvedilol and decreased by 3 meter in the placebo group (p=0.048). There was no difference between the groups on the 9-min treadmill test and in quality of life scores. Carvedilol was associated with greater improvement in NYHA class (p=0.014). Whereas the proportion of patients with NYHA class III or IV remains unchanged in the placebo group (from 58% to 51%), it decreased in the carvedilol treated patients (from 64% to 41%). A deterioration in NYHA class was observed in 3% of the carvedilol group vs 15% of the placebo group (p=0.001). Global assessment of disease severity by the patients and by the physicians revealed greater improvement with carvedilol than placebo. Left ventricular ejection fraction increased by 0.08 and 0.03 units with carvedilol and placebo therapy (p<0.001). 16.5% of the carvedilol-treated patients vs 25.5% of the placebo group had a cardiovascular hospitalization (p=0.06), and 4.5% vs 7.6% died (p=0.26). Death or cardiovascular hospitalization occurred in 19.6% of the carvedilol group vs 31.0% of the placebo group (p=0.029). The effects of carvedilol were similar in patients with ischemic or non-ischemic cardiomyopathy.

Conclusions

In patients with moderate to severe stable heart failure due to systolic dysfunction who are treated with diuretics, angiotensin converting enzyme inhibitors and digoxin, and can tolerate carvedilol treatment, carvedilol produces clinical benefits.

DiDi

Diltiazem in Dilated Cardiomyopathy

Title	Diltiazem improves cardiac function and exercise capacity in patients with idiopathic dilated cardiomyopathy. Results of the diltiazem in dilated cardiomyopathy trial.
Authors	Figulla HR, Gietzen F, Zeymer U, et al.
Reference	Circulation 1996;94:346-352.
Disease	Dilated cardiomyopathy.
Purpose	To evaluate whether diltiazem in addition to conventional therapy improves survival, hemodynamics, and well-being in patients with idiopathic dilated cardiomyopathy.
Design	Randomized, double blind, placebo-controlled, multicenter.
Patients	186 patients, 18-70 years old, with idiopathic dilated cardiomyopathy (LVEF<0.50). Patients with hypertension, 2nd or 3rd degree AV block, valvular or congenital heart disease, coronary artery disease, active myocarditis, insulin dependent diabetes, or systemic disease were excluded. Patients with previous treatment with any calcium antagonist or ß-blocker for >3 months were not included.
Follow-up	Coronary angiography with left heart catheterization, pulmonary artery catheterization at rest and during supine ergometry, 24 hour ambulatory ECG monitoring, echocardiography, radionuclide ventriculography, endomyocardial biopsy, plasma norepinephrine and ergorespirometry at baseline. Patients were followed every 6 months for 2 years.
Treatment regimen	Placebo or diltiazem started at 30 mgX3/d. Target dose was 90 mgX3/d or 60 mgX3/d (for patients weighing ≤50 kg).

Additional therapy

Any other calcium antagonist or ß blocker was prohibited. ACE inhibitors, digitalis, diuretics, and nitrates were prescribed as needed.

Results

33 patients dropped out of the study (13 receiving placebo and 20 receiving diltiazem). 24-month survival was 80.6% for the placebo vs 83.3% for the diltiazem group (p=0.78). Of the 153 patients that finished the protocol, 27 died or had a listing for heart transplantation (16 in the placebo and 11 in the diltiazem). The transplant listing-free survival was 85% for diltiazem vs 80% for the placebo (p=0.44). After 2 years, only the diltiazem group had an increase in cardiac index at rest (0.37±1.40 vs 0.33±1.14 L/min in the placebo, p=0.011), cardiac index at workload (0.57±1.52 vs 0.33±1.81 L/min, p=0.017), stroke volume index (8±24 vs 3±18 mL/m^2, p=0.003), and stroke work index (15±31 vs 5±20 g • min • m^{-2}, p=0.000), and decreased pulmonary artery pressure under workload (-5.2±12.2 vs -3.4±10.9 mmHg, p=0.007). Diltiazem increased exercise capacity (180±450 vs 60±325 W • min, p=0.002), and subjective well being (p=0.01). Adverse effects were minor and evenly distributed in both groups.

Conclusions

Diltiazem improves cardiac function, exercise capacity, and subjective status in patients with idiopathic dilated cardiomyopathy without deleterious effects on transplant listing-free survival.

PRAISE

Prospective Randomized Amlodipine Survival Evaluation trial

Title	Effect of amlodipine on morbidity and mortality in severe chronic heart failure.
Authors	Packer M, O'Connor CM, Ghali JK, et al.
Reference	N Engl J Med 1996;335:1107-1114.
Disease	Congestive Heart failure.
Purpose	To evaluate the long term effect of amlodipine, a calcium channel blocker, on mortality and morbidity in patients with advanced congestive heart failure.
Design	Randomized, double blind, placebo controlled, multicenter.
Patients	1153 patients with congestive heart failure (NYHA class IIIB or IV) and left ventricular ejection fraction <0.30, despite therapy with digoxin, diuretics and an angiotensin-converting-enzyme inhibitor. Patients with uncorrected primary valvular disease, active myocarditis, constrictive pericarditis, history of cardiac arrest or who had sustained ventricular fibrillation or tachycardia within the previous year, unstable angina or acute myocardial infarction within the previous month, cardiac revascularization or stroke within three months, severe concomitant disease, hypotension or hypertension, or serum creatinine >3.0 mg/dL were excluded.
Follow-up	6 to 33 months (median 13.8 months).
Treatment regimen	Randomization to amlodipine or placebo. The initial dose of amlodipine was 5 mg X1/d for two weeks and than increased to 10 mg/d.
Additional therapy	Diuretics, digoxin, and an angiotensin-converting-enzyme inhibitor. Nitrates were permitted, but other vasodilators, beta-blockers, calcium channel blockers and class IC antiarrhythmic agents were prohibited.

Prospective Randomized Amlodipine Survival Evaluation trial (continued)

Results

Of the patients with ischemic heart disease, 370 were assigned to placebo and 362 to amlodipine. Of the patients with nonischemic cardiomyopathy, 212 were assigned to placebo and 209 patients to amlodipine. A primary end point of the study (mortality from all causes or cardiovascular morbidity, defined as hospitalization for ≥24 hours for pulmonary edema, severe hypoperfusion, acute myoca.-dial infarction, or ventricular tachycardia/ fibrillation) was reached by 39% of the amlodipine-treated patients and in 42% of the placebo group. Amlodipine therapy was associated with insignificant risk reduction of primary end-points (9%; 95% CI 24% reduction to 10% increase; p=0.31). 33% vs 38% of the amlodipine and control groups died, respectively (16% risk reduction; 95% CI 31% reduction to 2% increase; p=0.07). Among patients with ischemic etiology, amlodipine therapy did not affect mortality or the combined end-point of mortality and cardiovascular morbidity. 45% of the patients in both groups had a fatal or non-fatal event, and 40% of the patients in both groups died. However, in patients with nonischemic cardiomyopathy amlodipine was associated with better outcome. Primary end-point was reached by 36.8% of the placebo, but in only 27.8% of the amlodipine group (31% risk reduction; 95% CI 2% to 51% reduction; p=0.04). Mortality was 34.9% vs 21.5% in the placebo and amlodipine group, respectively (46% risk reduction; 95% CI 21% to 63% reduction; p<0.001). Subgroup analysis revealed that amlodipine therapy was not associated with adverse effects in any of the subgroups. A favorable effect on survival was found only in patients without a history of angina. Total adverse effects that mandated discontinuation of double-blind therapy was comparable between the groups. However, peripheral edema (27% versus 18%, p<0.001) and pulmonary edema (15% versus 10%, p=0.01) occurred more frequently in the amlodipine group, while uncontrolled hypertension (2% versus <1%, p=0.03) and symptomatic cardiac ischemia (31% versus 25% among patients with ischemic heart disease, p=0.07) was more frequent in the placebo than amlodipine group. The frequencies of myocardial infarction, arrhythmias, and worsening of heart failure were similar.

Conclusions

Amlodipine was not associated with increased mortality and morbidity among patients with severe congestive heart failure. Amlodipine was associated with better outcome in patients with non-ischemic cardiomyopathy, whereas in patients with ischemic heart disease there was no difference in outcome.

SWORD

Survival With ORal D-sotalol

Title	a. The SWORD trial. Survival with oral d-sotalol in patients with left ventricular dysfunction after myocardial infarction: rationale, design and methods. b. Effect of d-sotalol on mortality in patients with left ventricular dysfunction after recent and remote myocardial infarction.
Authors	Waldo AL, Camm AJ, deRuyter H, et al.
Reference	a. Am J Cardiol 1995;75:1023-1027. b. Lancet 1996;348:7-12.
Disease	Congestive heart failure.
Purpose	To evaluate the effectiveness of d-sotalol, an antiarrhythmic agent with a pure potassium-channel-blocking effect, to reduce mortality in patients with previous myocardial infarction and left ventricular dysfunction.
Design	Randomized, double blind, placebo-controlled, multicenter.
Patients	3121 patients, age ≥18 years, with left ventricular ejection fraction of ≤40% and a recent (6-42 days) or a remote (>42 days) myocardial infarction and class II-III heart failure. Patients with unstable angina, class IV heart failure, history of life-threatening arrhythmia unrelated to a myocardial infarction, sick sinus syndrome or high-grade atrioventricular block, recent (<14 days) coronary angioplasty or coronary artery bypass surgery, electrolyte abnormalities, prolonged QT, renal failure, concomitant use of antiarrhythmic drugs were excluded.
Follow-up	Mean follow-up 148 days.

SWORD

Survival With ORal D-sotalol
(continued)

Treatment regimen	Randomization to oral d-sotalol 100 mgX2/d or placebo for 1 week. If the dose was tolerated and QTc<520 msec, the dose was increased to 200 mgX2/d. If QTc was >560 msec, the dose was reduced.
Additional therapy	β blockers, calcium channel blockers, digoxin, diuretics, nitrates, and angiotensin converting enzyme inhibitors were permitted.
Results	The trial was stopped prematurely after 3121 patients had been enrolled because of excess in mortality in the d-sotalol group. All causes mortality was 5.0% vs 3.1% in the d-sotalol and placebo group, respectively (relative risk (RR) 1.65; 95% CI 1.15 to 2.36; p=0.006), cardiac mortality was 4.7% vs 2.9%, respectively (RR 1.65; 95% CI 1.14 to 2.39; p=0.008), and presumed arrhythmic deaths 3.6% vs 2.0% (RR 1.77; 95% CI 1.15 to 2.74; p=0.008). Rates of non-fatal cardiac events were similar between the groups. The adverse effect associated with d-sotalol therapy was greater in patients with left ventricular ejection fraction of 31-40% than in those with ≤30% (RR 4.0 vs 1.2; p=0.007).
Conclusions	D-sotalol therapy in patients after myocardial infarction and a reduced left ventricular ejection fraction was associated with increased total and cardiac mortality, which was presumed primarily to be due to arrhythmic deaths

PICO

Pimobendan In Congestive heart failure

Title	Effect of pimobendan on exercise capacity in patients with heart failure: main results from the pimobendan in congestive heart failure (PICO) trial.
Authors	The Pimobendan in Congestive Heart Failure (PICO) Investigators.
Reference	Heart 1996;76:223-231.
Disease	Congestive heart failure.
Purpose	To assess the effects of pimobendan, a positive inotropic agent, on exercise capacity in patients with congestive heart failure.
Design	Randomized, double blind, placebo-controlled, multicenter.
Patients	317 patients, ≥18 years old, with stable chronic heart failure (NYHA class II-III), and left ventricular ejection fraction of ≤0.45. Patients with stenotic, obstructive, or infectious cardiac disease, exercise capacity limited by angina, on waiting list for transplantation, acute myocardial infarction, coronary revascularization, episodes of syncope or cardiac arrest within 3 months, AICD implantation, or severe concomitant disease were excluded. Patients in whom a first testing dose of pimobendan caused significant intolerance were excluded.
Follow-up	24 weeks of therapy with repeated exercise tests (efficacy phase). Clinical follow-up for a mean of 11 months.
Treatment regimen	Randomized to placebo or pimobendan 1.25 or 2.5 mg twice a day.

PICO

Pimobendan In Congestive heart failure
(continued)

Additional therapy

An angiotensin converting enzyme inhibitor and a diuretic were mandatory. Digitalis, nitrates, and molsidomine were permitted. Other inotropic agents, phosphodiesterase inhibitors, ibopamine, antiarrhythmic agents (except amiodarone), ß blockers, calcium antagonists, and other vasodilators were prohibited.

Results

Exercise duration on bicycle ergometry of the 2.5 mg/d pimobendan-treated patients was 13, 27, and 29 seconds longer than that of the placebo-treated patients, after 4, 12, and 24 weeks of therapy, respectively (p=0.03), and in the 5 mg/d treated patients it was 19, 17, and 28 seconds longer than that of the placebo group (p=0.05). After 24 weeks of therapy there was no difference in the percent of patients still alive and able to exercise to at least the baseline level (63% of the pimobendan group vs 59% of the placebo group; p=0.5). Pimobendan did not affect oxygen consumption, or quality of life (assessed by questionnaire). 4% of the placebo vs 10% of the pimobendan-treated patients did not worsen or die and were in better NYHA class at least once during follow-up than at baseline; p=0.06). Double blind therapy was stopped or reduced more often in the pimobendan than placebo treated group (p=0.04). All cause mortality after a mean of 11 months of follow-up was lower in the placebo group (10.8 per 100 person-years) than in the pimobendan treated patients (21.3 and 17.4 per 100 person-years in the 2.5 mg/d and 5 mg/d groups) (Hazard ratio of the pimobendan 2.5 mg/d 2.0; 95% CI 0.9 to 4.1; and that of the 5.0 mg/d 1.6; 95% CI 0.7 to 3.4). When both pimobendan groups were combined, the hazard ratio of death was 1.8 (95% CI 0.9 to 3.5) times higher than in the placebo group.

Conclusions

Pimobendan therapy in patients with congestive heart failure and left ventricular ejection fraction ≤0.45 was associated with an increase in exercise capacity. However, there was a trend towards an increased mortality in the treated patients.

DIG

The Digitalis Investigation Group study

Title	The effect of digoxin on mortality and morbidity in patients with heart failure.
Authors	The Digitalis Investigation Group.
Reference	N Engl J Med 1997;336:525-533.
Disease	Congestive heart failure
Purpose	To assess the effects of digoxin on morbidity and mortality in patients with heart failure and normal sinus rhythm.
Design	Randomized, double blind, placebo-controlled, multicenter.
Patients	6800 patients with left ventricular ejection fraction of ≤0.45 and 988 patients with left ventricular ejection fraction of >0.45. All patients had heart failure and were in sinus rhythm.
Follow-up	The mean duration of follow-up was 37 months (28 to 58 months).
Treatment regimen	Digoxin or placebo.
Additional therapy	Angiotensin-converting-enzyme inhibitors were encouraged. If patients remained symptomatic despite efforts to optimize other forms of therapy, open-label digoxin therapy was allowed and the study drug was discontinued.

DIG

The Digitalis Investigation Group study

(continued)

Results

In patients with ejection fraction ≤0.45, the mortality was similar (34.8% with digoxin and 35.1% with placebo. risk ratio 0.99; 95% CI 0.91-1.07, p=0.80). Cardiovascular mortality was similar (29.9% vs 29.5% in the digoxin and placebo group, respectively). There was a trend toward lower mortality ascribed to worsening of heart failure among the digoxin treated patients (11.6% vs 13.2%; risk ratio 0.88; 95% CI 0.77-1.01; p=0.06). Hospitalization rate due to cardiovascular reasons was lower in the digoxin treated group (49.9% vs 54.4%, risk ratio 0.87; 95% CI 0.81-0.93; p<0.001). Hospitalization rate due to worsening of heart failure was lower in the digoxin group (26.8% vs 34.7%, respectively; risk ratio 0.72; 95% CI 0.66-0.79; p<0.001).There was no significant difference between the two groups in hospitalization rate for ventricular arrhythmia or cardiac arrest (4.2% vs 4.3%). In all, 64.3% of the digoxin and 67.1% of the placebo group were hospitalized (risk ratio 0.92; 95% CI 0.87-0.98; p=0.006). There was no difference in hospitalization rate for myocardial infarction or unstable angina and for non-cardiovascular reasons. At one year, 85.6% and 82.9% of the digoxin and placebo treated patients were taking the study medication. At the final study visit, 70.8% of the surviving digoxin-treated patients were taking study medication and an additional 10.3% received open-label digoxin. In the placebo-group, 67.9% of the patients that were alive were taking placebo and 15.6% received open-label digoxin. In the cohort of patients with left ventricular ejection fraction >0.45, mortality was 23.4% in both groups. The combined end-point of death or hospitalization for worsening of heart failure occurred less in the digoxin-treated patients (risk ratio 0.82; 95% CI 0.63-1.07).

Conclusions

Digoxin therapy in patients with heart failure and left ventricular ejection fraction ≤0.45 was associated with lower rates of overall hospitalization and hospitalization due worsening of heart failure. There was no difference in mortality and occurrence of myocardial ischemia or arrhythmia between the digoxin and placebo groups.

ELITE

Evaluation of Losartan In The Elderly

Title

Randomised trial of losartan versus captopril in patients over 65 with heart failure (Evaluation of Losartan in the Elderly study, ELITE).

Authors

Pitt B, Martinez FA, Meurers GG, et al.

Reference

Lancet 1997;349:747-752.

Disease

Congestive heart failure.

Purpose

To compare the efficacy and safety of losartan (a specific angiotensin II receptor blocker) and captopril (an angiotensin converting enzyme inhibitor) in the treatment of elderly patients with heart failure.

Patients

722 patients, ≥65 years old, with symptomatic heart failure (NYHA class II-IV), left ventricular ejection fraction ≤0.40, and no history of prior angiotensin converting enzyme inhibitor therapy. Patients with systolic blood pressure <90 mmHg or diastolic blood pressure >95 mmHg, significant obstructive valvular heart disease, symptomatic arrhythmias, pericarditis or myocarditis, PTCA within 72h, CABG within 2 weeks, ICD within 2 weeks, likelihood for cardiac surgery during the study period, acute myocardial infarction within 72 h, unstable angina within 3 months, stable angina, stroke or transient ischemic attack within 3 months, concomitant severe disease, creatinine ≥2.5 mg/dl, anemia, leukopenia, and electrolyte disturbances were excluded.

Follow-up

48 weeks

Treatment regimen

A 2-week placebo run-in phase, and then randomization to captopril (6.25 mg-50 mgX3/d) plus placebo losartan, or placebo captopril plus losartan (12.5-50 mgX1/d).

Additional therapy Treatment with all other cardiovascular medications (except open-label angiotensin converting enzyme inhibitors) was permitted

Results 352 patients were randomized to losartan and 370 to captopril. Persisting increases in serum creatinine (≥0.3 mg/dl) occurred in 10.5% in each group (risk reduction 2%; 95% CI -51% to 36%; p=0.63). Death and/or admissions for heart failure occurred in 9.4% in the losartan group vs 13.2% in the captopril group (risk reduction 32%; 95% CI -4% to 55%; p=0.075). Mortality was 4.8% in the losartan group vs 8.7% in the captopril group (risk reduction 46%; 95% CI 5% to 69%; p=0.035). Sudden death occurred in 1.4% vs 3.8%, respectively (risk reduction 64%; 95% CI 3% to 86%). The cumulative survival curves separated early and remained separated throughout the study. 22.2% of the losartan group vs 29.7% of the captopril group were admitted to the hospital for any reason (risk reduction 26%; 95% CI 5% to 43%; p=0.014). However, there was no difference in admission for heart failure (5.7% in each group; p=0.89). NYHA class improved in both treatment groups. The percentage of patients in NYHA class I or II was increased form 66% at baseline to 80% at the end of the study in the losartan group, and from 64% to 81% in the captopril group. 18.5% of the losartan group vs 30% of the captopril group discontinued the study medication or died (p≤0.001). 12.2% vs 20.8% of the patients, respectively, discontinued the study medication because of adverse effects p≤0.002). Cough leading to discontinuation of therapy was reported in 0 vs 3.8%, respectively. Persistent (≥0.5 mmol/L) increases in serum potassium was observed in 18.8% of the losartan group vs 22.7% of the captopril group (p=0.069).

Conclusions Losartan therapy was associated with lower mortality and hospitalization rate than captopril therapy in elderly patients with symptomatic heart failure. Losartan was better tolerated than captopril.

7. Lipid Lowering Studies

POSCH

Program On the Surgical Control of the Hyperlipidemias

Title	Effect of partial ileal bypass surgery on mortality and morbidity from coronary heart disease in patients with hypercholesterolemia. Report of the Program on the Surgical control of the hyperlipidemias (POSCH).
Authors	Buchwald H, Varco RL, Matts JP, et al.
Reference	N Engl J Med 1990;323:946-955.
Disease	Hyperlipidemia, coronary artery disease.
Purpose	To evaluate whether cholesterol lowering inducea by the partial ileal bypass operation would reduce mortality or morbidity due to coronary heart disease.
Design	Randomized, open label.
Patients	838 patients, 30-64 years of age, 6-60 montns after a single myocardial infarction with total plasma cholesterol> 5.69 mmol/l or LDL cholesterol> 3.62 mmol/l. Patients with hypertension, diabetes mellitus, or obesity were excluded
Follow-up	7-14.8 years (mean 9.7 years).
Treatment regimen	Partial ileal bypass of either the distal 200 cm or 1/3 of the small intestine, whichever was greater.
Additional therapy	American Heart Association Phase II diet. Hypocholesterolemic medications were discontinued.

Results

Five years after randomization the surgical group had lower total plasma cholesterol (4.71±0.91 vs. 6.14±0.89 mmol/l; $p<0.0001$) and LDL-cholesterol (2.68±0.78 vs. 4.30±0.89 mmol/l; $p<0.0001$); while HDL-cholesterol was higher (1.08±0.26 vs. 1.04±0.25 mmol/l; $p=0.02$). There was a trend towards lower overall mortality and mortality due to coronary artery disease in the surgical group, however without statistical significance. The combined end point of cardiovascular death or nonfatal myocardial infarction was 35% lower in the surgical group (82 vs. 125 events; $p<0.001$). The surgical group had less disease progression on follow-up angiograms ($p<0.001$ at 5 and 7 years). During follow-up, 52 and 137 patients of the surgical and control groups underwent coronary artery bypass grafting surgery ($p<0.0001$), while 15 and 33 of the surgical and control group patients underwent angioplasty ($p=0.005$).

Conclusions

Partial ileal bypass surgery induced a sustained reduction in plasma cholesterol levels and reduced the morbidity due to coronary artery disease.

FATS

Familial Atherosclerosis Treatment Study

Title	Regression of coronary artery disease as a result of intensive lipid lowering therapy in men with high levels of apolipoprotein B.
Authors	Brown G, Alberts JJ, Fisher LD, et al.
Reference	N Engl J Med 1990;323:1289-1298.
Disease	Hyperlipidemia, coronary artery disease.
Purpose	To assess the effect of intensive lipid-lowering therapy on coronary atherosclerosis among high risk men.
Design	Randomized, double blind, placebo (or colestipol) controlled, multicenter.
Patients	146 men, ≤62 years of age, with plasma levels of apolipoprotein ß ≥125 mg/dl, documented coronary artery disease (≥1 lesion of ≥50% stenosis, or ≥3 lesions of ≥30% stenosis), and a positive family history of vascular disease.
Follow-up	Clinical evaluation, plasma lipid levels, and coronary angiography at baseline and at 30 months.
Treatment regimen	1. Lovastatin 20 mg X2/d, and colestipol 10gX3/d. 2. Niacin 1gX4/d, and colestipol 10gX3/d. 3. Placebo or colestipol (if LDL cholesterol exceeded the 90th percentile for age).
Additional therapy	American Heart Association Phase I and II diet.

Results

The levels of LDL and HDL cholesterol changed only slightly in the control group (mean change -7% and +5%, respectively). However they were improved with the lovastatin+colestipol (-46% and +15%) or niacin+colestipol (-32% and +43%) arms. In the control group 46% of the patients had definite lesion progression, while 11% had regression. Progression was observed in only 21% and 25% of the lovastatin+ colestipol and niacin+colestipol patients, while regression was observed in 32% and 39%, respectively (p for trend=0.005). Multivariate regression analysis revealed that reduction in the apolipoprotein ß levels, and in systolic blood pressure, and an increase in HDL cholesterol were associated with regression of coronary lesions. Death, myocardial infarction, or revascularization due to worsening symptoms occurred in 10 of the 52 patients with conventional therapy, as compared to 3 of 46 and 2 of 48 of the lovastatin+colestipol and niacin+colestipol treated patients (p=0.01). Overall, intensive lipid-lowering therapy reduces the incidence of clinical events by 73% (95% CI 23-90%).

Conclusions

In men with coronary artery disease who are at high risk, intensive lipid-lowering therapy reduced the frequency of progression and increases regression of atherosclerotic coronary lesions, and reduced the incidence of cardiovascular events.

EXCEL

Expanded Clinical Evaluation of Lovastatin

Title	a. Expanded clinical evaluation of lovastatin (EXCEL) study: design and patient characteristics of a double-blind, placebo-controlled study in patients with moderate hypercholesterolemia. b. Expanded clinical evaluation of lovastatin (EXCEL) study results. I. Efficacy in modifying plasma lipoproteins and adverse event profile in 8245 patients with moderate hypercholesterolemia. c. Expanded clinical evaluation of lovastatin (EXCEL) study results: III. Efficacy in modifying lipoproteins and implications for managing patients with moderate hypercholesterolemia. d. Expanded clinical evaluation of lovastatin (EXCEL) study results: IV. Additional perspectives on the tolerability of lovastatin.
Authors	a-c. Bradford RH, Shear CL, Chremos AN, et al. d. Dujovne CA, Chermos AN, Pool JL, et al.
Reference	a. Am J Cardiol 1990;66:44B-55B. b. Arch Intern Med 1991;151:43-49. c. Am J Med 1991;91(suppl 1B):18S-24S. d. Am J Med 1991;91(suppl 1B):25S-30S.
Disease	Hypercholesterolemia.
Purpose	To evaluate dose-response relation of lovastatin in lipid/lipoprotein modifying efficacy and of drug related adverse effects in patients with moderate hypercholesterolemia.
Design	Randomized, double blind, multicenter.
Patients	8245 patients, age 18-70 years, with primary type II hyperlipidemia (fasting total plasma cholesterol 6.21-7.76 mmol/l, LDL cholesterol ≥4.14 mmol/l, and triglyceride <3.95 mmol/l). Patients with diabetes mellitus requiring medications, secondary hypercholesterolemia and premenopausal women were excluded.

EXCEL

Expanded Clinical Evaluation of Lovastatin

(continued)

Follow-up	48 weeks.
Treatment regimen	One of the following regimens for 48 weeks: 1. lovastatin 20 mg X1/d; 2. lovastatin 40 mg X1/d; 3. lovastatin 20mg X2/d; 4. lovastatin 40mg X2/d; and 5. placebo.
Additional therapy	American Heart Association phase I diet.
Results	Lovastatin therapy resulted in a sustained, dose-related decrease of total cholesterol (-17%, -22%, -24%, and -29% for groups 1-4, while it increased by +0.7% in the placebo group, p<0.001 for dose trend), of LDL-cholesterol (-24%, -30%, -34%, and -40% for groups 1-4, while it increased by +0.4% in the placebo group, p<0.001 for dose trend) and of triglyceride (-10%, -14%, -16%, and -19%, respectively, while in the placebo it increased by 3.6%, p<0.001 for dose trend). HDL cholesterol increased by 6.6%, 7.2%, 8.6%. and 9.5%, respectively, while in the placebo it increased in only 2.0%. (p<0.001 for dose trend). Patients withdrawal due to adverse effects occurred in 6% of the placebo and 7-9% of the lovastatin groups. Increases in serum transaminase occurred in 0.1%, 0.1%, 0.9%, 0.9%, and 1.5% of groups 1-5, p<0.001 for trend). Myopathy was rare.
Conclusions	Lovastatin is a safe and highly effective and well tolerated therapy for hypercholesterolemia.

MAAS

Multicentre Anti-Atheroma Study

Title	Effect of simvastatin on coronary atheroma: the Multicentre Anti-Atheroma Study (MAAS).
Authors	MAAS Investigators.
Reference	Lancet 1994;344:633-638.
Disease	Coronary artery disease.
Purpose	To evaluate the effects of simvastatin on coronary atheroma in patients with moderate hypercholesterolemia and coronary artery disease.
Design	Randomized, double blind, placebo controlled, multicenter.
Patients	381 patients, age 30-67 years, with documented coronary artery disease, serum cholesterol 5.5-8.0 mmol/l and triglyceride <4.0 mmol/l. Patients with unstable angina or myocardial infarction within 6 weeks, angioplasty or surgery within 3 months, treated diabetes mellitus, or patients with congestive heart failure or ejection fraction <30% were excluded.
Follow-up	Clinical follow-up for 4 years. Coronary angiography before therapy was started and after 2 and 4 years.
Treatment regimen	Simvastatin 20 mg/d or placebo.
Additional therapy	Lipid lowering diet.

MAAS

Multicentre Anti-Atheroma Study

(continued)

Results

Patients receiving simvastatin had 23% reduction of serum cholesterol, 31% reduction of LDL cholesterol, and a 9% increase in HDL cholesterol compared with placebo after 4 years. 345 patients had repeated angiograms after 4 years. Mean luminal diameter was reduced by 0.08±0.26 mm vs 0.02±0.23 mm in the placebo and simvastatin groups (treatment effect 0.06, 95% CI 0.02-0.10), and minimal luminal diameter was reduced by 0.13±0.27 mm vs 0.04±0.25 mm (treatment effect 0.08, 95% CI 0.03-0.14) (combined p=0.006). Diameter stenosis was increased by 3.6±9.0% vs 1.0±7.9%, respectively (treatment effect -2.6%, 95% CI -4.4% to -0.8%). The beneficial effect of simvastatin was observed regardless of the initial diameter stenosis. Angiographic progression occurred in 32.3% vs 23.0% of the placebo and simvastatin groups, and regression in 12.0% vs 18.6%, respectively (combined p=0.02). New lesions developed in 3.7% vs 2.0% of the segments studied, respectively. There was no difference in clinical outcome. However, more patients in the placebo than simvastatin group (34 vs 23 patients) underwent coronary revascularization.

Conclusions

Simvastatin 20 mg/d reduced hyperlipidemia and slowed the progression of diffuse and focal coronary artery disease.

4S

Scandinavian Simvastatin Survival Study

Title	a. Randomized trial of cholesterol lowering in 4444 patients with coronary heart disease: the Scandinavian Simvastatin Survival Study (4S). b. Baseline serum cholesterol and treatment effect in the Scandinavian Simvastatin Survival Study (4S). c. Reducing the risk of coronary events: evidence from the Scandinavian Simvastatin Survival Study (4S).
Authors	a+b. Scandinavian Simvastatin Survival Study Group. c. Kjekshus J, Pedersen TR, for the Scandinavian Simvastatin Survival Study Group
Reference	a. Lancet 1994;344:1383-1389. b. Lancet 1995;345:1274-1275. c. Am J Cardiol 1995;76:64C-68C.
Disease	Coronary artery disease, hyperlipidemia.
Purpose	To assess the effect of simvastatin therapy on mortality and morbidity of patients with coronary artery disease and serum cholesterol 5.5-8.0 mmol/l.
Design	Randomized, double blind, placebo controlled, multicenter.
Patients	4444 patients, aged 35-70 years, with a history of angina pectoris or myocardial infarction, and serum cholesterol 5.5-8.0 mmol/l, and serum triglyceride ≤2.5 mmol/l. Premenopausal women and patients with secondary hypercholesterolemia were excluded. Patients with myocardial infarction within 6 months, congestive heart failure, planned coronary artery surgery or angioplasty were not included.
Follow-up	Clinical follow-up for 4.9-6.3 years (median 5.4 years).

4S

Scandinavian Simvastatin Survival Study

(continued)

Treatment regimen Simvastatin 20 mg/d or placebo. If serum cholesterol did not reach the target range of 3.0-5.2 mmol/l by simvastatin 20 mg/d, the dose was increased to 40 mg/d, or decreased to 10 mg/d.

Additional therapy Dietary advice.

Results Lipid concentrations changed only little in the placebo group, whereas simvastatin resulted in -25%, -35%, +8%, and -10% change from baseline of total-, LDL-, and HDL-cholesterol, and triglycerides. After 1 year, 72% of the simvastatin group had achieved total cholesterol <5.2 mmol/l. During the follow-up mortality was 12% in the placebo and 8% in the simvastatin group (RR 0.70, 95% CI 0.58-0.85, p=0.0003). The Kaplan-Meier 6-year probability of survival was 87.7% in the placebo vs 91.3% in the simvastatin group. Coronary mortality was 8.5% vs 5.0%, respectively (RR 0.58, 95% CI 0.46-0.73). There was no difference in noncardiovascular death. 28% of the placebo and 19% of the simvastatin group had one or more major coronary events (coronary death, myocardial infarction, or resuscitated cardiac arrest (RR 0.66, 95% CI 0.59-0.75, p<0.00001). The relative risk of having any coronary event in the simvastatin group was 0.73 (95% CI 0.66-0.80, p<0.00001). Simvastatin also reduced the risk of undergoing coronary artery bypass surgery or angioplasty (RR 0.63, 95% CI 0.54-0.74, p<0.00001). The overall rates of adverse effects were not different between the groups. Simvastatin significantly reduced the risk of major coronary events in all quartiles of baseline total, HDL, and LDL cholesterol, by a similar amount in each quartile.

Conclusions Long term therapy with simvastatin is safe and effective in improvement of survival and reduction of the rate of coronary events.

PLAC I and II

Pravastatin Limitation of Atherosclerosis in the Coronary Arteries

Title	a. Design and recruitment in the United States of a multicenter quantitative angiographic trial of pravastatin to limit atherosclerosis in the coronary arteries (PLAC I). b. Pravastatin, lipids, and atherosclerosis in the carotid arteries (PLAC-II). c. Reduction in coronary events during treatment with pravastatin.
Authors	a. Pitt B, Ellis SG, Mancini GBJ, et al. b. Crouse JR III, Byington RP, Bond MG, et al. c. Furberg CD, Pitt B, Byington RP, et al.
Reference	a. Am J Cardiol 1993;72:31-35. b. Am J Cardiol 1995;75:455-459. c. Am J Cardiol 1995;76:60C-63C.
Disease	Hyperlipidemia.
Purpose	To assess the effects of pravastatin on progression and regression of coronary artery disease in patients with moderate hypercholesterolemia.
Design	Randomized, double blind, placebo controlled, multicenter.
Patients	559 patients (PLAC I: 408 patients, age ≤75 years, with documented ≥1 stenosis ≥50% in a major epicardial coronary artery, LDL cholesterol 130-189 mg/dl, and triglycerides ≤350 mg/dl. Patients with secondary hyperlipidemia, diabetes mellitus, congestive heart failure, and other serious concomitant diseases were excluded. PLAC II: 151 patients with coronary artery disease and extracranial carotid lesion. Same criteria as above.).
Follow-up	Clinical follow-up for 3 years. Coronary angiography at baseline and after 36 months (PLAC I).

PLAC I and II

Pravastatin Limitation of Atherosclerosis in the Coronary Arteries

(continued)

Treatment regimen	Pravastatin 40 mg X1/d or placebo for 3 years in PLAC-I, 20-40 mg/d in PLAC-II.
Additional therapy	Patients whose LDL cholesterol remained ≥190 mg/dl received cholestyramine, and then 5-10 mg open-label pravastatin or placebo. If these measures failed, the patient was withdrawn from the study.
Results	The incidence of coronary events was 4.0%/year in the placebo vs 1.8%/year in the pravastatin patients (55% risk reduction, 95% CI 19-79%, p=0.014). A similar effect was seen in patients <65 years and ≥65 years of age. 11 patients vs 7 patients in the placebo and pravastatin groups died (40% risk reduction, 95% CI -65% to 85%, p=0.31). Nonfatal myocardial infarction occurred in 24 patients of the placebo vs 9 of the pravastatin group (67% risk reduction, 95% CI 32%-88%, p=0.006). The angiographic results have not been published yet.
Conclusions	Pravastatin therapy was associated with reduction of clinical events in coronary patients with mild to moderate hyperlipidemia.

WOSCOPS

Prevention of Coronary Heart Disease With Pravastatin in Men With Hypercholesterolemia. The West of Scotland Coronary Prevention Study

Title	Prevention of coronary heart disease with pravastatin in men with hypercholesterolemia.
Authors	Shepherd J, Cobbe SM, Ford I, et al.
Reference	N Engl L Med 1995;333:1301-1307.
Disease	Hypercholesterolemia.
Purpose	To assess whether pravastatin therapy reduces the incidence of acute myocardial infarction and mortality from coronary heart disease in hypercholesterolemic men without a history of prior myocardial infarction.
Design	Randomized, double-blind, placebo controlled, multicenter.
Patients	6595 men, 45-64 years of age, with fasting LDL cholesterol >252 mg per deciliter before diet and >155 mg per deciliter after 4 weeks of diet. None of the patients had a history of prior myocardial infarction. 78% of the patients were ex- or current smokers and 5% had angina pectoris.
Follow-up	The average follow-up was 4.9 years (32,216 subject-years of follow-up).
Treatment regimen	Pravastatin (40 mg/d) or placebo.

WOSCOPS

Prevention of Coronary Heart Disease With Pravastatin in Men With Hypercholesterolemia. The West of Scotland Coronary Prevention Study

(continued)

Results

Compared to baseline values pravastatin reduced plasma total cholesterol levels by 20% and LDL-cholesterol by 26%, whereas no such changes were observed in the placebo-treated group. Pravastatin reduced coronary events by 31% (95% CI 17-43%; p<0.001). There were 174 (5.5%) and 248 (7.9%) coronary events in the pravastatin and control group, respectively. Pravastatin reduced the risk for nonfatal infarction by 31% (4.6% versus 6.5%; p<0.001; 95% CI 15-45%), and the risk for death from all cardiovascular causes by 32% (1.6 versus 2.3%; p=0.033; 95% CI 3-53%). There was no increase in mortality from noncardiovascular causes.

Conclusions

Primary prevention in moderately hypercholesterolemic men with 5 years Pravastatin therapy reduced the incidence of myocardial infarction and death from cardiovascular causes. No excess of noncardiovascular death was observed.

REGRESS

The Regression Growth Evaluation Statin Study

Title	a. Effects of lipid lowering by pravastatin on progression and regression of coronary artery disease in symptomatic men with normal to moderately elevated serum cholesterol levels. The regression Growth Evaluation Statin Study (REGRESS). b. Reduction of transient myocardial ischemia with pravastatin in addition to the conventional treatment in patients with angina pectoris.
Authors	a. Jukema JW, Bruschke AVG, van Boven AJ, et al. b. van Boven AJ, Jukema JW, Zwinderman AH, et al.
Reference	a. Circulation 1995;91:2528-2540. b. Circulation 1996;94:1503-1505.
Disease	Hyperlipidemia, coronary artery disease.
Purpose	To evaluate whether 2 years of statin therapy will affect the progression of coronary artery disease and clinical outcome of patients with coronary artery disease who have normal to moderately elevated plasma cholesterol levels.
Design	Randomized, double blind, placebo controlled, multicenter.
Patients	a. 885 men with serum cholesterol 4-8 mmol/L and ≥1 coronary lesion with ≥50% of luminal narrowing. b. 768 men with stable angina pectoris, with serum cholesterol 4-8 mmol/L and ≥1 coronary lesion with ≥50% of luminal narrowing.
Follow-up	a. Clinical evaluation and repeated angiography after 2 years. b. Ambulatory holter ECG monitoring before randomization, and after intervention (in patients that underwent CABG or PTCA) or after 2 years (in patients treated medically).

REGRESS

The Regression Growth Evaluation Statin Study

(continued)

Treatment regimen Pravastatin 40 mg/d or placebo.

Additional therapy Dietary advice. Cholestyramine for patients with cholesterol >8.0 mmol/L on repeated assessments. Routine antianginal therapy.

Results a. 778 (88%) had an evaluable final coronary angiography. Mean segment diameter decreased 0.10 mm and 0.06 mm in the placebo and pravastatin groups (mean difference 0.04 mm, 95% CI 0.01-0.07 mm, p=0.19). The median minimum obstruction diameter decreased 0.09 and 0.03 mm, respectively (difference of the medians 0.06 mm, 95% CI 0.02-0.08 mm, p=0.001). After 2 years 89% of the pravastatin and 81% of the placebo treated patients were without new cardiovascular events (p=0.002).
b. In the pravastatin-assigned patients, transient myocardial ischemia was detected at baseline in 28% and after treatment in 19%. In the placebo-treated patients it was found in 20% at baseline and 23% at follow-up (odds ratio 0.62; 95% CI 0.41 to 0.93; p=0.021). The number of ischemic episodes per ambulatory ECG monitoring was reduced at follow-up by 0.53±0.25 episodes in the placebo group and by 1.23±0.25 episodes in the pravastatin group (p=0.047). Ischemic burden (the product of duration of ischemia in minutes multiplied by ST segment depression in mm) decreased from 41±5 to 22±5 mm • min in the pravastatin treated patients (p=0.0058), and from 34±6 to 26±4 mm • min in the placebo group (p=0.24). After adjustment for other independent risk factors, the effect of pravastatin on reduction of ischemia remained significant (odds ratio 0.45; 95% CI 0.22 to 0.91; p=0.026).

Conclusions a. 2 years of pravastatin therapy, in men with coronary artery disease and normal to moderately elevated cholesterol levels, resulted in less progression of coronary atherosclerosis and fewer new cardiovascular events.
b. Pravastatin ameliorated transient myocardial ischemia in patients with coronary artery disease and optimal antianginal therapy.

CARE

Cholesterol And Recurrent Events

Title	The effect of pravastatin on coronary events after myocardial infarction in patients with average cholesterol levels.
Authors	Sacks FM, Pfeffer MA, Moye LA, et al.
Reference	1. Am J Cardiol 1991;68:1436-1446. 2. Am J Cardiol 1995;75:621-623. 3. Am J Cardiol 1995;76:98C-106C. 4. N Engl J Med 1996;335:1001-1009.
Disease	Coronary artery disease, myocardial infarction.
Purpose	To evaluate the effectiveness of lowering blood cholesterol levels with pravastatin in patients after myocardial infarction and its effect on subsequent cardiac events.
Design	Randomized, double blind, placebo-controlled, multicenter.
Patients	4159 patients, 21-75 years old, who have experienced myocardial infarction 3-20 months before randomization, and had plasma total cholesterol <240 mg/dl, LDL cholesterol 115-174 mg/dl, triglycerides <350 mg/dl, fasting glucose levels ≤ 220 mg/dl, left ventricular ejection fraction ≥25%, and no symptomatic congestive heart failure.
Follow-up	Median follow-up 5 years (4-6.2 years).
Treatment regimen	Pravastatin 40 mg/d or placebo. For patients with LDL cholesterol >175 mg/dl at follow-up, dietary counseling and then cholestyramine.
Results	Pravastatin therapy lowered the mean LDL cholesterol of 139 mg/dl by 32% and maintained mean levels of 98 mg/dl. During follow-up LDL cholesterol was 28% lower, total cholesterol was 20% lower, HDL 5% higher, and triglycerides level 14% lower in the pravastatin than placebo group (p< 0.001 for all comparisons). Primary endpoints (death from coronary artery disease or non-fatal myocardial infarction)

occurred in 13.2% vs. 10.2% in the placebo and pravastatin group, respectively (risk reduction 24%; 95% CI 9 to 36%; p=0.003). Cardiovascular death occurred in 5.7% in the placebo vs. 4.6% in the pravastatin group (risk reduction 20%; 95% CI -5 to 39%; p=0.10), and non-fatal myocardial infarction occurred in 8.3% vs. 6.5%, respectively (risk reduction 23%; 95% CI 4 to 39%; p=0.02). However, total mortality was comparable (9.4% vs. 8.6% in the placebo and pravastatin group, respectively; 9% risk reduction; 95% CI -12 to 26%; p=0.37). There was no difference in mortality from non-cardiovascular causes. The risk of myocardial infarction was 25% lower in the pravastatin group (7.5% vs. 10.0%; 95% CI 8 to 39%; p=0.006). The rate of coronary artery bypass surgery or PTCA was lower in the pravastatin group (14.1% vs. 18.8%; risk reduction 27%; 95% CI 15 to 37%; p<0.001). The pravastatin group had also a 31% lower incidence of stroke (2.6% vs. 3.8%; 95% CI 3 to 52%; p=0.03). There was also a trend toward less unstable angina in the pravastatin group (15.2% vs. 17.3%; risk reduction 13%; 95% CI -1 to 25%; p=0.07). The effect of pravastatin was greater among women then among men (46% vs. 20% risk reduction for women and men respectively). Patients with baseline LDL cholesterol >150 mg/dl had a 35% reduction in major coronary events, as compared with a 26% reduction in those with baseline LDL cholesterol of 125 to 150 mg/dl, and a 3% increase in those with baseline levels < 125 mg/dl (p=0.03 for the interaction between baseline LDL cholesterol level and risk reduction). The overall incidence of fatal or nonfatal cancer was comparable (161 in the placebo vs 172 in the pravastatin group). However, breast cancer occurred in 1 patient in the placebo and in 12 in the pravastatin group (p=0.002). Of the 12 cases in the pravastatin group, 3 occurred in patients who had previously had breast cancer. There was no other significant differences between the groups in the occurrence of other types of cancer.

Conclusions Pravastatin therapy lowered cardiac mortality, the need for revascularization, and occurrence of stroke in both men and women with coronary artery disease, plasma total cholesterol of <240 mg per deciliter and plasma LDL cholesterol >125 mg per deciliter. In this study, no reduction in event rate was found in patients with LDL cholesterol <125 mg per deciliter. There was no reduction in overall mortality

8. Arrhythmia

CAST

Cardiac Arrhythmia Suppression Trial

Title	a. Preliminary report: effect of encainide and flecainide on mortality in a randomized trial of arrhythmia suppression after myocardial infarction. b. Mortality and morbidity in patients receiving encainide, flecainide, or placebo. The Cardiac Arrhythmia Suppression Trial c. Events in the Cardiac Arrhythmia Suppression Trial (CAST): mortality in the entire population enrolled. d. Events in the Cardiac Arrhythmia Suppression Trial (CAST): mortality in patients surviving open label titration but not randomized to double-blind therapy. e. Association between ease of suppression of ventricular arrhythmia and survival.
Authors	a. The CAST Investigators. b. Echt DS, Leibson PR, Mitchell LB, et al. c. Epstein AE, Bigger JT Jr, Wyse DG, et al. d. Wyse DG, Hallstrom A, McBride R, et al. e. Goldstein S, Brooks MM, Ledingham R, et al.
Reference	a. N Engl J Med 1989;321:406-412. b. N Engl J Med 1991;324:781-788. c. J Am Coll Cardiol 1991;18:14-19. d. J Am Coll Cardiol 1991;18:20-28. e. Circulation 1995;91:79-83.
Disease	Ventricular arrhythmia, coronary artery disease.
Purpose	To evaluate whether suppression of asymptomatic or mildly symptomatic ventricular arrhythmias in patients after myocardial infarction would reduce mortality from arrhythmia.
Design	Randomized, open label (titration phase), double blind (main phase), placebo controlled, multicenter.
Patients	2309 patients, 6 d to 2 years after myocardial infarction, with ≥6 PVCs per h, and left ventricular ejection fraction of ≤0.55 for patients with infarction within 90 days and ≤0.40 for patients with infarction 90 d to 2 years before randomization. Patients with ventricular arrhythmias that caused severe symptoms (such as presyncope or syncope) were excluded.

CAST

Cardiac Arrhythmia Suppression Trial

(continued)

Follow-up

An average of 9.7 months.

Treatment regimen

An open label titration phase (average 15 d), during which up to 3 drugs (encainide, flecainide and moricizine) at 2 oral doses were tested. This phase was terminated as soon as suppression of ≥80% of the PVCs and ≥90% suppression of nonsustained ventricular tachycardia was detected by 24 h ambulatory ECG monitoring 4-10 d after each dose was begun. Flecainide was not used in patients with ejection fraction <0.30. In patients with ejection fraction ≥0.30, moricizine was used as a second drug. Patients whose arrhythmia worsened or who were intolerant were not included in the main phase. In the main phase patients were randomized to receive either the active drug, that had suppressed the arrhythmia, or placebo.

Results

1727 patients (75%) had initial suppression of their arrhythmia and were included in the main phase. 1498 patients were assigned to flecainide, encainide or placebo. After an average of 10 months total mortality was 7.7% in the encainide/flecainide groups vs 3.0% in the placebo (relative risk 2.5, 95% CI 1.6-4.5). The relative risks for death from any cause for encainide and flecainide considered separately were not different (2.7 vs 2.2 compared to placebo). Death from arrhythmia was more common in the encainide/flecainide groups (4.5%) than placebo (1.2%, relative risk 3.6, 95% CI 1.7-8.5, p=0.0004). The relative risk for encainide was 3.4 and for flecainide 4.4, compared with placebo. The relative risk for death or cardiac arrest with resuscitation was 2.38 (95% CI 1.59-3.57). Subgroup analyses revealed that in every subgroup tested, flecainide and encainide were associated with increased total mortality and arrhythmic death. The mortality in the placebo-treated patients was lower than expected. This was probably due to selection bias of including only patients whose arrhythmias were suppressable in the titration phase. Non-randomized patients had more extensive coronary disease and experienced higher mortality and arrhythmic events than the randomized placebo group.

Conclusions

Encainide and flecainide were associated with increased death rate due to arrhythmia and acute myocardial infarction complicated by shock in patients after acute myocardial infarction with asymptomatic ventricular arrhythmias, even though these drugs were effective in suppression of the arrhythmia.

BASIS

Basel Antiarrhythmic Study of Infarct Survival

Title	a. Effect of antiarrhythmic therapy on mortality in survivors of myocardial infarction with asymptomatic complex ventricular arrhythmias: Basel Antiarrhythmic Study of Infarct Survival (BASIS). b. Long-term benefit of 1-year amiodarone treatment for persistent complex ventricular arrhythmias after myocardial infarction.
Authors	a. Burkart F, Pfisterer M, Kiowski W, et al. b. Pfisterer ME, Kiowski W, Brunner H, et al.
Reference	a. J Am Coll Cardiol 1990;16:1711-1718. b. Circulation 1993;87:309-311.
Disease	Arrhythmia, acute myocardial infarction.
Purpose	To evaluate the effects of prophylactic antiarrhythmic treatment in survivors of myocardial infarction with persisting asymptomatic complex arrhythmias.
Design	Randomized, 3 centers.
Patients	312 patients, <71 years old, who survived acute myocardial infarction and had asymptomoatic complex ventricular ectopic activity on a 24 h ECG recording 24 h after discontinuation of all antiarrhythmic medications.
Follow-up	a. Clinical evaluation and 24 h ECG monitoring at baseline and after 3, 6 and 12 months. b. 55-125 months (mean 72 months).

BASIS

Basel Antiarrhythmic Study of Infarct Survival

(continued)

Treatment regimen	Patients were randomized to either: 1. Individualized antiarrhythmic drugs guided by continuous ECG monitoring (quinidine and mexiletine as first line drugs and ajmaline, disopyramide, flecainide, propafenone or sotalol as second line drugs). If none of these drugs suppressed the arrhythmias- amiodarone was given. 2. Low dose amiodarone. 1g/d for 5 days followed by 200 mg/d. If symptomatic arrhythmias developed, the therapy was changed and the patients were considered to be treatment deviators. Treatment was continued for 1 year. 3. Control without prophylactic antiarrhythmic drug. If symptoms occurred, antiarrhythmic medications were given, and they were considered as treatment deviators.
Additional therapy	No limitations on other non-antiarrhythmic medications.
Results	a. During 1 year follow-up, 10%, 5.1%, and 13.2% of groups 1, 2, and 3 died (61% reduction of mortality by amiodarone vs control ($p=0.048$). After exclusion of non-cardiac mortality, amiodarone was still associated with 55% reduction of mortality. Sudden death or sustained ventricular tachycardia or fibrillation occurred in 5.1% of the amiodarone and 16.7% of the control group ($p<0.01$). The effect of individualized therapy (group 1) was less marked (40% reduction, p=NS). b. The probability of death after 84 months (Kaplan Meier) was 30% for amiodarone and 45% for control patients ($p=0.03$). However, this was entirely due to the first year amiodarone effect. A similar effect was observed regarding cardiac death ($p=0.047$).
Conclusions	Low dose amiodarone decreased mortality during the first year after acute myocardial infarction in asymptomatic patients with persistent complex ventricular arrhythmias. The beneficial effect of amiodarone lasted several years after discontinuation of amiodarone

CASCADE

Cardiac Arrest in Seattle: Conventional Versus Amiodarone Drug Evaluation

Title	a. Cardiac arrest in Seattle: conventional versus amiodarone drug evaluation (the CASCADE study). b. the CASCADE study: randomized antiarrhythmic drug therapy in survivors of cardiac arrest in Seattle.
Authors	a. The CASCADE Investigators. b. Greene HL, for the CASCADE Investigators.
Reference	a. Am J Cardiol 1991;67:578-584. b. Am J Cardiol 1993;72:70F-74F.
Disease	Ventricular fibrillation.
Purpose	To evaluate the efficacy of empiric amiodarone therapy and electrophysiologic testing and ambulatory ECG monitoring guided drug therapy in survivors of out-of-hospital ventricular fibrillation.
Design	Randomized, open label, multicenter.
Patients	228 patients who survived an episode of out-of-hospital ventricular fibrillation that was not associated with Q wave infarction. Only patients who were considered high-risk for recurrence were included.
Follow-up	Up to 6 years.
Treatment regimen	Amiodarone or electrophysiologic testing and ambulatory ECG monitoring guided conventional drug therapy.
Additional therapy	Approximately 50% of all patients received an implanted defibrillator (Since 1988).

CASCADE

Cardiac Arrest in Seattle: Conventional Versus Amiodarone Drug Evaluation

(continued)

Results

Of the 115 patients randomized to conventional therapy 33 received quinidine, 26 procainamide, 12 received flecainide, and 17 combination therapy. 82% and 69% of the amiodarone and conventional therapy groups were free from either cardiac death, resuscitated VF, or syncopal shocks from implanted defibrillator after 2 years. The corresponding numbers for 4 and 6 years are 66% vs 52% and 53% vs 40%, in the amiodarone and conventional therapy groups, respectively (p=0.007). 83% vs 78%, 65% vs 62%, and 58% vs 37% of the patients were still alive after 2, 4, and 6 years. 105 patients had automatic implantable defibrillators. 38% of the amiodarone and 60% of the conventional therapy experienced shock from the defibrillator (p=0.032). However, 29% of the amiodarone and only 17% of the conventional therapy group stopped their medications. Possible pulmonary toxicity was diagnosed in 6% of the patients over 12 months and 10% over 3 years. Thyroid dysfunction was relatively common (22.1%) in the amiodarone group.

Conclusions

Although amiodarone was associated with mild reduction of mortality, overall mortality remained high, and side effects were common.

CAST-2

Cardiac Arrhythmia Suppression Trial-2

Title	a. The Cardiac Arrhythmia Supression Trial: first CAST.. then CAST-II. b. Effect of the antiarrhythmic agent moricizine on survival after myocardial infarction.
Authors	a. Greene HL, Roden DM, Katz RJ, et al. b. The Cardiac Arrhythmia Suppression Trial II investigators.
Reference	a. J Am Coll Cardiol 1992;19:894-898. b. N Engl J Med 1992;327:227-233.
Disease	Ventricular arrhythmia, coronary artery disease.
Purpose	To evaluate whether suppression of asymptomatic or mildly symptomatic ventricular premature depolarizations by moricizine would decrease mortality in patients after myocardial infarction.
Design	Randomized, double blind, placebo controlled, multicenter.
Patients	Patients, 6-90 d after myocardial infarction, with ≥6 PVCs per h, and left ventricular ejection fraction of ≤0.40. Patients with ventricular arrhythmias that caused severe symptoms (such as presyncope or syncope), or runs ≥30 seconds at a rate of ≥120 bpm were excluded. 1325 patients (10 patients were included in CAST-I) were included in the short term trial and 1374 patients (536 patients were included in CAST-I) in the long-term trial.
Follow-up	Short-term protocol: 2 weeks. Long-term protocol: a mean of 18 months.

Treatment regimen

Short-term protocol: moricizine 200 mg X3/d for 14 d vs placebo or no therapy. Long-term protocol: titration phase of moricizine started with 200 mg X3/d and increased to 250 mg X3/d and then to 300 mg X3/d until arrhythmia was suppressed or adverse effects occurred. Only patients in whom suppression of ≥80% of the PVCs and ≥90% suppression of nonsustained ventricular tachycardia was detected by 24 h ambulatory ECG monitoring were entered into the long-term protocol.

Results

CAST-II was stopped early because moricizine therapy was associated with excess mortality in the first 14-day phase. The rate of death or resuscitated cardiac arrest was 2.6% (17 of 665 patients) of the moricizine group vs 0.5% (3 of 660 patients) of the no therapy group (adjusted $p<0.01$, relative risk 5.6, 95% CI 1.7-19.1). Other adverse effects such as recurrent myocardial infarction, new or worsened heart failure, and proarrhythmia tended to be higher in the moricizine group. Arrhythmia suppression was achieved in 1155 patients (87.2%) who were included in the long-term phase. During a mean follow-up of 18 months 8.4% of the moricizine vs 7.3% of the placebo treated group died or had cardiac arrests due to arrhythmias ($p=0.4$). The 2 year survival rate was 81.7% in the moricizine vs 85.6% in the placebo. Nonfatal adverse effects were more common with moricizine ($p=0.03$).

Conclusions

Moricizine was effective in suppression of asymptomatic or mildly symptomatic ventricular arrhythmias in patients after myocardial infarction. However, therapy with moricizine was associated with increased mortality in the short protocol and no beneficial effect in the long-term protocol.

ESVEM

The Electrophysiologic Study Versus Electrocardiographic Monitoring

Title a. The ESVEM Trial: electrophysiologic study versus electrocardiographic monitoring for selection of antiarrhythmic therapy of ventricular tachyarrhythmias.
b. Determinants of predicted efficacy of antiarrhythmic drugs in the electrophysiologic study versus electrocardiographic monitoring trial.
c. A comparison of electrophysiologic testing with holter monitoring to predict antiarrhythmic-drug efficacy for ventricular tachyarrhythmias.
d. A comparison of seven antiarrhythmic drugs in patients with ventricular tachyarrhythmias.
e. Cost of initial therapy in the electrophysiological study versus ECG monitoring trial (ESVEM).
f. Significance and incidence of concordance of drug efficacy predictions by holter monitoring and electrophysiological study in the ESVEM Trial.

Authors a.+b. The ESVEM Investigators.
c.+d. Mason JW, for the ESVEM Investigators.
e. Omioigui NA, Marcus FI, Mason JW, et al.
f. Reiter MJ, Mann DE, Reiffel JE, et al.

Reference a. Circulation 1989;79:1354-1360.
b. Circulation 1993;87:323-329.
c. N Engl J Med 1993;329:445-451
d. N Engl J Med 1993;329:452-458.
e. Circulation 1995;91:1070-1076.
f. Circulation 1995;91:1988-1995.

Disease Ventricular tachyarrhythmias.

Purpose To compare the efficacy and accuracy of electrophysiologic study (EPS) versus ambulatory electrocardiographic holter monitoring (HM) for prediction of antiarrhythmic drug efficacy in patients with aborted sudden death or sustained ventricular tachyarrhythmias.

Design Randomized, open label, multicenter.

ESVEM

The Electrophysiologic Study Versus Electrocardiographic Monitoring

(continued)

Patients	486 patients who had been resuscitated from sudden death, or had documented sustained ventricular tachycardia or unmonitored syncope (with subsequent EPS demonstration inducible sustained monomorphic ventricular tachycardia) were screened. Only patients with ≥10 PVCs/h during 48 h HM and reproducibly inducible sustained ventricular tachyarrhythmias at EPS were included.
Follow-up	6.2 years.
Treatment regimen	Patients were randomized to serial drug evaluation by HM and exercise test or by EPS. Patients underwent testing of up to 6 drugs until one or none was predicted to be effective: imipramine, mexiletine, procainamide, quinidine, sotalol, pirmenol, and propafenone. Drugs were tested in random order. Patients were discharged from the hospital with a predicted effective drug. Subjects in whom no drug was effective were withdrawn from the study.
Results	Efficacy predictions were achieved in 45% of the EPS and 77% in the HM arms ($p<0.001$). Ejection fraction of <0.25 and presence of coronary artery disease were negative correlates ($p<0.10$) of drug efficacy prediction in the EPS arm. In the HM arm, only ejection fraction correlated with efficacy, although with only marginal significance ($p=0.11$). A multivariate model selected assessment by HM and higher ejection fraction as independent predictors ($p<0.05$) of drug efficacy. The drug evaluation process required an actuarial median time of 25 days in the EPS vs 10 days in the HM arms ($p<0.0001$). There was no significant difference between the EPS and HM arms in the actuarial probabilities of either death or recurrence of arrhythmia. Patients randomized to EPS had higher mean charge for evaluation ($42,002 vs $29,970, $p=0.0015$) and more drug trials (3.0 vs 2.1, $p=0.0001$). In the EPS group, the percentage of patients who had predictions of drug efficacy was higher with sotalol (35%) than with any other drugs (26%-10%, $p<0.001$). There was no significant difference among the drugs in the HM group. The least adverse effects was noted with sotalol (16% vs 23%-43% with the other drugs). The patients that received sotalol had the lowest actuarial probability of recurrence of ventricular arrhythmia (RR 0.43, 95%

CI 0.29-0.62, p<0.001), death from any cause (RR 0.50, 95% CI 0.30-0.80, p=0.004), cardiac death (RR 0.50, 95% CI 0.28-0.90, p=0.02), or arrhythmic death (RR 0.50, 95% CI 0.26-0.96, p=0.04). At the time of the first drug trial in the EPS group, HM and EPS were concordant in predicting efficacy in 23% and in predicting inefficiency in 23%. In 54% of the patients there was discordance between HP and EPS. At the time EPS predicted efficacy, 68 of the 100 patients also had suppression of arrhythmias in HM. Rates of arrhythmia recurrence or mortality were similar among patients with suppression of arrhythmias on both HM and EPS, compared with those who had suppression on EPS alone. There was no significant difference in outcome between the patients with suppression on both HM and EPS and those with suppression on the HM arm.

Conclusions Drug efficacy predictions are achieved more frequently and faster with HM than EPS strategy. However, there was no significant difference in the success of drug therapy as selected by either EPS or HM. Sotalol was more effective than the other 6 drugs in preventing death and recurrence of ventricular arrhythmia, and was associated with less adverse effects than the other medications. There is frequent discordance in prediction of drug efficacy between HM and EPS. However, suppression of ventricular arrhythmias on both tests did not predict better outcome.

MADIT

The Multicenter Automatic Defibrillator Implantation Trial

Title	Improved survival with an implanted defibrillator in patients with coronary disease at high risk for ventricular arrhythmia.
Authors	Moss AJ, Hall WJ, Cannom DS, et al.
Reference	N Engl J Med 1996;335:1933-1940.
Disease	Coronary artery disease, arrhythmia.
Purpose	To assess whether prophylactic implantation of cardioverter-defibrillator, as compared with conventional medical therapy, would decrease mortality in patients with prior myocardial infarction, low ejection fraction, and episodes of asymptomatic unsustained ventricular tachycardia.
Design	Randomized, multicenter.
Patients	196 patients of either sex, 25 to 80 years old, with myocardial infarction >3 weeks before entry, documented episode of asymptomatic, nonsustained ventricular tachycardia (3 to 30 ventricular ectopic beats at a rate >120 per min), and left ventricular ejection fraction ≤0.35. Patients in NYHA class IV, indication for revascularization, previous cardiac arrest or symptomatic ventricular tachycardia, CABG within 2 months or PTCA within 3 months, advanced cerebrovascular disease, and serious noncardiac medical condition were not included. Eligible patients underwent electrophysiologic study, and only patients with reproducibly induced ventricular tachycardia or fibrillation that was not suppressed by procainamide or an equivalent drug were included.
Follow-up	Average follow-up 27 months (range <1 month to 61 months).

MADIT

The Multicenter Automatic Defibrillator Implantation Trial

(continued)

Treatment regimen

Within 30 days after the electrophysiologic study, patients were randomized to implantation of defibrillator or conventional medical therapy. The choice of medical therapy, including whether to use antiarrhythmic agents, was made by the patient's physician. The first 98 patients were randomized to medical therapy (n=53) or transthoracic defibrillator (n=45), and the last 98 patients to medical therapy (n=48) or nonthoracotomy defibrillator implantation with transvenous leads (n=50).

Results

The baseline characteristics of the defibrillator and medical therapy groups were similar. Eleven patients in the medical therapy group received a defibrillator during the follow-up period, and 5 patients assigned to defibrillator never received a defibrillator. There were no operative deaths. There were 15 deaths in the defibrillator group and 39 deaths in the medical therapy group (hazard ratio 0.46; 95% CI 0.26 to 0.82; p=0.009). There were 11 deaths from cardiac causes in the defibrillator group vs 27 in the medical therapy group. Both defibrillator types, with transthoracic and with intravenous leads were equally effective (ratio of the hazard ratios 0.86; p=0.78). There was no evidence that ß blockers, amiodarone, or other antiarrhythmic drugs had an influence on the hazard ratio. However, the power of the analysis for the drug interactions with hazard ratio is limited, due to small number of treated patients.

Conclusions

In patients with prior myocardial infarction, reduced left ventricular ejection fraction, and asymptomatic nonsustained ventricular tachycardia, who had reproducible sustained ventricular arrhythmia during electrophysiologic study that was not suppressible by intravenous antiarrhythmic drug, prophylactic implantation of defibrillator improved survival as compared with conventional medical therapy.

9. Anticoagulation for Atrial Fibrillation

AFASAK

Aspirin vs Warfarin in Atrial Fibrillation

Title	Placebo-controlled, randomized trial of warfarin and aspirin for prevention of thromboembolic complications in chronic atrial fibrillation. The Copenhagen AFASAK study.
Authors	Petersen P, Boysen G, Godtfredsen J, et al.
Reference	Lancet 1989;I:175-179.
Disease	Atrial fibrillation.
Purpose	To evaluate the effects of low dose aspirin and warfarin anticoagulation on the incidence of thromboembolic events in patients with chronic non-rheumatic atrial fibrillation.
Design	Randomized, open label (warfarin vs no-warfarin), double blind in the group of no-warfarin (aspirin vs placebo), two centers.
Patients	1007 patients, ≥18 years old with chronic atrial fibrillation. Patients with previous anticoagulation therapy >6 months, cerebrovascular event within 1 month, severe hypertension, alcoholism, valve replacement, rheumatic heart disease, or with contraindication to aspirin or warfarin were excluded.
Follow-up	2 years.
Treatment regimen	Warfarin (open label), target INR was 2.8-4.2. Aspirin 75 mg/d or placebo.

Results

Patients on warfarin were within INR 2.8-4.2 for 42% of the time. 26% of the time the INR was <2.4. Thromboembolic complications occurred in 1.5% of the warfarin, 6.0% in the aspirin, and 6.3% of the control group ($p<0.05$). The yearly incidence of thromboembolic events was 2.0% on warfarin and 5.5% on either aspirin or placebo. Vascular death occurred in 0.9%, 3.6%, and 4.5% of the warfarin, aspirin and placebo groups ($p<0.02$). 6.3% of the warfarin patients had non-fatal bleeding, while only 0.6% and 0 of the aspirin and placebo patients had bleeding.

Conclusions

Chronic anticoagulation with warfarin, but not with low-dose aspirin, reduced vascular mortality and thromboembolic complications in patients with chronic nonrheumatic atrial fibrillation.

SPAF

Stroke Prevention in Atrial Fibrillation

Title	a. Preliminary report of the stroke prevention in atrial fibrillation study. b. Stroke prevention in atrial fibrillation study. Final results.
Authors	SPAF Investigators.
Reference	a. N Engl J Med 1990;322:863-868. b. Circulation 1991;84:527-539.
Disease	Atrial fibrillation.
Purpose	To determine the efficacy of warfarin and aspirin for primary prevention of ischemic stroke and systemic embolism in patients with non-rheumatic atrial fibrillation.
Design	Randomized, open label (warfarin), double blind (aspirin vs placebo), multicenter.
Patients	1330 patients with chronic or paroxysmal atrial fibrillation, without prosthetic heart valve or rheumatic mitral stenosis. Patients with congestive heart failure were excluded. 627 patients were eligible to receive warfarin (group 1), and 703 patients were not eligible (group 2).
Follow-up	a. An average of 1.13 years. b. An average of 1.3 years.
Treatment regimen	Group 1. warfarin vs aspirin 325 mg/d or placebo. Target INR for warfarin 2.0-4.5. Group 2. aspirin 325 mg/d vs placebo.

SPAF

Stroke Prevention in Atrial Fibrillation

(continued)

Results	a. The overall primary events (ischemic stroke and embolism) rate was 1.6% per year in the patients who received either aspirin or warfarin, and 8.3% per year in the placebo treated patients in group 1 (risk reduction 81%, 95% CI 56-91%, p<0.00005). Total primary end points occurred in 3.2% and 6.3% of the aspirin and placebo treated patients (group 1+2)(risk reduction 49% (15-69%), p=0.014). On the basis of these results, the placebo arm was discontinued by the safety committee. b. Warfarin reduced the risk of primary events by 67% (2.3% vs 7.4% per year, 95% CI 27-85%, p=0.01). Aspirin reduced the risk of primary events by 42% (3.6% vs 6.3%, 95% CI 9-63%, p=0.02). Primary events or death were reduced by 58% (95% CI 20-78%, p=0.01) by warfarin and 32% (95% CI 7-50%, p=0.02) by aspirin. The risk of significant bleeding was 1.5%, 1.4%, and 1.6% per year in the warfarin, aspirin, and placebo, respectively.
Conclusions	Aspirin and warfarin are both effective in prevention of ischemic stroke and systemic embolism in patients with non-rheumatic atrial fibrillation.

BAATAF

Boston Area Anticoagulation Trial for Atrial Fibrillation

Title	The effect of low-dose warfarin on the risk of stroke in patients with nonrheumatic atrial fibrillation.
Authors	The Boston Area Anticoagulation Trial for Atrial Fibrillation Investigators.
Reference	N Engl J Med 1990;323:1505-1511.
Disease	Atrial fibrillation.
Purpose	To assess the efficacy of low-dose warfarin therapy in preventing stroke in patients with nonrheumatic atrial fibrillation.
Design	Randomized, open label, multicenter.
Patients	420 patients with chronic or paroxysmal atrial fibrillation without mitral stenosis. Patients with left ventricular thrombus, aneurysm, prosthetic heart valve, severe heart failure, transient ischemic attack or stroke within 6 months, or clear indication or contraindications to anticoagulant therapy were excluded.
Follow-up	Clinical follow-up up to 4.5 years (mean 2.2 years).
Treatment regimen	Warfarin (target range for prothrombin-time ratio 1.2-1.5X control value (INR 1.5-2.7), or no treatment.
Additional therapy	Aspirin therapy was not allowed in the anticoagulation group. Aspirin was permitted in the control group.

BAATAF

Boston Area Anticoagulation Trial for Atrial Fibrillation

(continued)

Results

Prothrombin time in the warfarin group was in the target range 83% of the time. Only 10% of the patients discontinued warfarin permanently. There were 2 strokes in the warfarin and 13 in the control groups (p=0.0022);(incidence of 0.41%/year vs 2.98%/year (incidence ratio 0.14, 95% CI 0.04-0.49. Two and 1 patients in the warfarin and control group had major bleeding. There was no statistical significant difference in the occurrence of minor bleeding. Total mortality was 11 and 26 patients in the warfarin and control patients (RR 0.38, 95% CI 0.17-0.82, p=0.005). The same trend was seen for cardiac and non-cardiac mortality. Patients with paroxysmal and chronic atrial fibrillation had similar risk of stroke.

Conclusions

Long term low dose warfarin therapy was associated with reduced mortality and prevention of stroke in patients with atrial fibrillation not associated with mitral stenosis.

CAFA

Canadian Atrial Fibrillation Anticoagulation

Title	Canadian Atrial Fibrillation Anticoagulation (CAFA) study.
Authors	Connolly SJ, Laupacis A, Gent M, et al.
Reference	J Am Coll Cardiol 1991;18:349-355.
Disease	Atrial fibrillation.
Purpose	To assess the efficacy and safety of warfarin therapy for nonrheumatic atrial fibrillation.
Design	Randomized, double blind, placebo controlled, multicenter.
Patients	378 patients, ≥19 years of age, with paroxysmal recurrent or chronic atrial fibrillation, without mitral stenosis or mitral or aortic prosthetic valves. Patients with clear indications or contraindications to anticoagulation therapy, stroke or transient ischemic attack within 1 year, myocardial infarction within 1 month, uncontrolled hypertension, or antiplatelet therapy were excluded.
Follow-up	Clinical follow-up for up to 2.75 years (mean 15.2 months).
Treatment regimen	Warfarin or placebo. Target INR for warfarin was 2-3.
Additional therapy	Aspirin or antiplatelet therapy was not advised.

CAFA

Canadian Atrial Fibrillation Anticoagulation

(continued)

Results

Early permanent discontinuation of the therapy, not due to primary outcome event, occurred in 26.2% of the warfarin and 22.5% of the placebo group. The estimated percent of days during which the INR was 2-3 was 43.7%. The ratio was bellow the target in 39.6% of the days. The annual rate of major bleeding was 0.5% in the placebo and 2.5% in the warfarin group. Minor bleeding occurred in 9.4% and 16% of the patients, respectively. The annual rate of ischemic nonlacunar stroke, systemic embolization, or intracranial or fatal hemorrhage was 3.5% and 5.2% in the warfarin and placebo groups (risk reduction 37%, 95% CI -63.5% to 75.5%, p=0.17).

Conclusions

Chronic anticoagulation therapy is relatively safe and effective therapy for reduction the risks of stroke and death in patients with nonrheumatic atrial fibrillation. This study was stopped prematurely due to the results of the AFASAK and SPAF studies.

SPINAF

Stroke Prevention in Nonrheumatic Atrial Fibrillation

Title	Warfarin in the prevention of stroke associated with non-rheumatic atrial fibrillation.
Authors	Ezekowitz MD, Bridgers SL, James KE, et al.
Reference	N Engl J Med 1992;327:1406-1412.
Disease	Atrial fibrillation.
Purpose	To evaluate whether low-intensity anticoagulation will reduce the risk of stroke among patients with non rheumatic atrial fibrillation.
Design	Randomized, double blind, placebo controlled, multicenter.
Patients	525 males, no age limitation, with atrial fibrillation and no echocardiographic evidence of rheumatic heart disease.
Follow-up	Up to 3 years (an average of 1.7 years).
Treatment regimen	Sodium warfarin or placebo. Target INR 1.4-2.8.
Additional therapy	Aspirin and other anti-inflammatory drugs were not permitted.

SPINAF

Stroke Prevention in Nonrheumatic Atrial Fibrillation

(continued)

Results

Patients assigned to warfarin had their INR within the target range 56% of the time. Among patients with no previous stroke, cerebral infarction occurred at a rate of 4.3% per year in the placebo vs 0.9% per year in the warfarin group (risk reduction of 0.79, 95% CI 0.52-0.90, p=0.001). The annual event rate among the 228 patients over 70 years of age was 4.8% vs 0.9%, respectively (risk reduction 0.79, 95% CI 0.34-0.93, p=0.02). Only 1 nonfatal cerebral hemorrhage occurred in a patient that received warfarin. Major hemorrhages occurred in 0.9% vs 1.3% in the placebo and warfarin no previous stroke groups (risk reduction -0.53, 95% CI -4.22 to 0.55, p=0.54). Mortality of patients without prior stroke was 5.0% in the placebo vs 3.3% in the warfarin group (risk reduction 0.31, 95% CI -0.29 to 0.63, p=0.19). In patients with prior stroke, cerebral infarction occurred in 4 of the 25 patients in the placebo and in 2 of the 21 patients in the warfarin group (risk reduction 0.40, 95% CI -1.66 to 0.87, p=0.63).

Conclusions

Low intensity anticoagulation with warfarin reduced the rate of cerebral infarction in patients with nonrheumatic atrial fibrillation, without association with excess risk of bleeding.

EAFT

The European Atrial Fibrillation Trial

Title	a. Secondary prevention in non-rheumatic atrial fibrillation after transient ischaemic attack or minor stroke. b. Optimal oral anticoagulant therapy in patients with non-rheumatic atrial fibrillation and recent cerebral ischemia.
Authors	The European Atrial Fibrillation Trial Study Group.
Reference	a. Lancet 1993;342:1255-1262. b. N Engl J Med 1995;333:5-10.
Disease	Atrial fibrillation.
Purpose	a. To evaluate the effectiveness of oral anticoagulant therapy and oral aspirin for secondary prevention in patients with nonrheumatic atrial fibrillation and recent transient ischemic attack or minor ischemic stroke. b. To determine the optimal intensity of anticoagulation for secondary prevention in patients with nonrheumatic atrial fibrillation and recent transient ischemic attack or minor ischemic stroke.
Design	Randomized, open label (oral anticoagulant), double blind (aspirin vs placebo), multicenter.
Patients	a. Group 1: 669 patients, >25 years old, with chronic or paroxysmal non-rheumatic atrial fibrillation and recent (<3 months) minor ischemic stroke or transient ischemic attack randomized to anticoagulant, aspirin or placebo. Group 2: 338 patients with the same clinical characteristics but with contraindication to oral anticoagulants randomized to aspirin or placebo. b. 214 patients with nonrheumatic atrial fibrillation and a recent episode of minor cerebral ischemia who received anticoagulant therapy.
Follow-up	Mean follow-up 2.3 years.

EAFT

The European Atrial Fibrillation Trial

(continued)

Treatment regimen

1. Oral anticoagulant (open label).
2. Aspirin 300 mg/d or placebo (double blind).

Results

a. Group 1. The annual rate of events (vascular death, stroke, myocardial infarction, and embolism) was 8% in patients assigned to anticoagulants and 17% in the placebo-treated (Hazard ratio 0.53, 95% CI 0.36-0.79). The risk of stroke was reduced from 12% to 4% per year (hazard ratio 0.34, 95% CI 0.20-0.57). Group 1+2: The annual incidence of outcome events was 15% in the aspirin vs 19% in the placebo (hazard ratio 0.83, 95% CI 0.65-1.05). The hazard ratio for stroke of aspirin vs placebo was 0.86 (95% CI 0.64-1.15). Anticoagulation was better than aspirin (hazard ratio 0.60, 95% CI 0.41-0.87; p=0.008).
b. The optimal anticoagulation that results in the lower rate of bleeding and ischemic episodes was of INR 2.0-3.9. Most major bleedings occurred when INR was ≥5.0.

Conclusions

a. Oral anticoagulant are a safe and effective therapy for secondary prevention. Aspirin is less effective than anticoagulants.
b. The target value for INR should be 3.0. Values <2.0 and >5.0 should be avoided.

SPAF-2

Stroke in Atrial Fibrillation II Study

Authors	Stroke Prevention in Atrial Fibrillation Investigators.
Title	Warfarin versus aspirin for prevention of thromboembolism in atrial fibrillation: stroke prevention in atrial fibrillation II study.
Reference	Lancet 1994;343:687-691.
Disease	Atrial fibrillation.
Purpose	To compare the efficacy of aspirin and warfarin for prevention of stroke and systemic embolism in patients with nonrheumatic atrial fibrillation.
Study Design	Randomized, multicenter.
Follow-up	Mean 2.3 years.
Treatment regimen	Warfarin (target prothrombin time ratio 1.3-1.8; INR 2.0-4.5) or aspirin 325 mg/d.
Patients	1100 patients (715 patients ≤75 years old and 385 patients >75 years old) with atrial fibrillation in the previous 12 months. Patients with prosthetic valves, mitral stenosis, or indication or contraindications to aspirin or warfarin were excluded. Patients <60 years old with lone atrial fibrillation and those with ischemic stroke or transient ischemic attack within 2 years were excluded.

SPAF-2

Stroke in Atrial Fibrillation II Study

(continued)

Results

In patients ≤75 years old primary events (ischemic stroke or systemic embolism) occurred at a rate of 1.3% per year in the warfarin group vs 1.9% in the aspirin group (RR 0.67, 95% CI 0.34-1.3, p=0.24). The absolute rate of primary events in low-risk younger patients (without hypertension, heart failure, or previous thromboembolism) was 0.5% on aspirin vs 1.0% on warfarin. Among older patients, the primary event rate was 3.6% per year with warfarin vs 4.8% with aspirin (RR 0.73, 95% CI 0.37-1.5, p=0.39). There was no statistically significant difference in mortality, or occurrence of all strokes with residual deficit between the aspirin and warfarin treated patients in both the ≤75 and >75 years old cohorts. In patients ≤75 years old rates of major hemorrhage were 0.9% per year with aspirin vs 1.7% per year with warfarin (p=0.17). For older patients the rates were 1.6% vs 4.2%, respectively (p=0.04).

Conclusions

Warfarin may be more effective than aspirin for prevention of ischemic stroke or systemic embolism in patients with nonrheumatic atrial fibrillation. However, the absolute reduction in total stroke rate is small. Younger patients without risk factors had a low rate of stroke when treated with aspirin. The risk was higher for older patients, irrespective of which agent was used.

Optimal Oral Anticoagulant Therapy in Patients With Mechanical Heart Valves

Title	Optimal oral anticoagulant therapy in patients with mechanical heart valves.
Authors	Cannegieter SC, Rosendaal FR, Wintzen AR, et al.
Reference	N Engl J Med 1995;333:11-17.
Disease	Mechanical heart valves.
Purpose	To determine the optimal intensity of anticoagulation in patients with mechanical heart valves.
Design	Events that occurred during a period of endocarditis were excluded.
Patients	1608 patients with mechanical valves.
Follow-up	up to 6 years (6475 patient-years).
Treatment regimen	Phenprocoumon or acenocoumarol.
Results	The optimal intensity of anticoagulant therapy is that associated with the lowest incidence of both thromboembolic and bleeding events. This level has been achieved with an INR values of 2.5-4.9. At this level of INR the incidence of all adverse events was 2 per 100 patient-years (95% CI 1.0-3.8). The incidence rose sharply to 7.5 per 100 patient-year when INR was 2.0-2.4 (95% CI 3.6-12.6), and to 4.8 per 100 patient-year (95% CI 2.6-7.7) when the INR rose to 5.0-5.5. When INR was ≥6.5, the incidence was 75 per 100 patient-year (95% CI 54-101).
Conclusions	The intensity of anticoagulation for patients with prosthetic mechanical valves is optimal when the INR is 2.5-4.9. A target INR of 3.0-4.0 is recommended.

SPAF III

Stroke Prevention in Atrial Fibrillation III

Title	Adjusted-dose warfarin versus low-intensity, fixed-dose warfarin plus aspirin for high-risk patients with atrial fibrillation: Stroke Prevention in Atrial Fibrillation III randomised clinical trial.
Authors	Stroke Prevention in Atrial Fibrillation Investigators.
Reference	Lancet 1996;348:633-638.
Disease	Atrial Fibrillation.
Purpose	To compare the efficacy of low-intensity fixed-dose warfarin plus aspirin with conventional adjusted-dose warfarin in patients with atrial fibrillation at high risk of stroke.
Design	Randomized, multicenter.
Patients	1044 patients with atrial fibrillation. In addition, patients had to have at least one of the following four risk factors: 1. Recent congestive heart failure or left ventricular systolic dysfunction, 2. Systolic blood pressure >160 mmHg, 3. Prior ischemic stroke, transient ischemic attack or systemic embolism >30 days prior to entry, or 4. Being a women >75 years old. Patients with prosthetic heart valves, mitral stenosis, recent pulmonary embolism, other conditions that needed anticoagulation therapy, contraindication to aspirin or warfarin. or regular use of non-steroidal anti-inflammatory drugs were excluded.
Follow-up	The trial was terminated prematurely after a mean follow-up of 1.1 years (range 0 to 2.5 years).
Treatment regimen	Randomization to either the combination therapy (warfarin 0.5 to 3.0 mg/d to raise INR to 1.2-1.5 on 2 successive measurements and aspirin 325 mg/d) or adjusted-dose warfarin (target INR 2.0-3.0).

SPAF III

Stroke Prevention in Atrial Fibrillation III

(continued)

Results

Withdrawal of assigned therapy unrelated to primary or secondary events occurred at a rate of 8.2% per year in the combination therapy group and 5.6% in the adjusted dose group ($p=0.13$). The mean INR was 1.3 vs 2.4 in the combination therapy and adjusted-dose groups . During the study period, 54% of the INRs in the combination therapy treated patients were 1.2 to 1.5 and 34% were <1.2. Among patients treated with adjusted dose warfarin, 61% of the INRs were within the therapeutic range 2.0 to 3.0, 25% were below this range. Ischemic stroke and systemic embolism occurred at a rate of 7.9% per year vs 1.9% per year in the combination therapy and adjusted dose group, respectively (absolute rate difference 6.0%; 95% CI 3.4 % to 8.6%; $p<0.0001$). The annual rates of disabling or fatal stroke (5.6% vs 1.7%; $p=0.0007$) and of stroke, systemic embolism or vascular death (11.8% vs 6.4%; $p=0.002$) were higher in the combination therapy group. By analysis restricted to patients taking assigned therapy, the relative risk reduction by adjusted dose vs combination therapy was 77% for stroke or systemic embolism ($p<0.0001$) and 48% for stroke, systemic embolism or vascular death ($p=0.002$). Rates of major bleeding were comparable (2.4% per year vs 2.1% per year in the combination therapy and adjusted dose group, respectively).

Conclusions

The efficacy of low-intensity fixed dose warfarin plus aspirin in preventing stroke, systemic embolism or vascular death in patients with atrial fibrillation at high-risk for thromboembolism is inferior to the conventional adjusted dose warfarin therapy.

10. Coronary Artery Disease, Atherosclerosis- Prevention of Progression

INTACT

International Nifedipine Trial on Antiatherosclerotic Therapy

Title	Retardation of angiographic progression of coronary artery disease by nifedipine. Results of the International Nifedipine Trial on Antiatherosclerotic Therapy (INTACT).
Authors	Lichtlen PR, Hugenholtz PG, Rafflenbeul W, et al.
Reference	Lancet 1990;335:1109-1113.
Disease	Coronary artery disease.
Purpose	To evaluate the effects of 3 years of nifedipine therapy on progression of coronary artery disease and formation of new lesions.
Design	Randomized, double blind, placebo controlled, multicenter.
Patients	348 patients, <65 years old, with mild or single vessel coronary artery disease. Patients with multivessel disease, ejection fraction <40%, mandatory therapy with calcium channel blockers, or prior therapy with calcium channel blockers >6 months were excluded.
Follow-up	Clinical follow-up and repeated angiography after 36 months.
Treatment regimen	Placebo or nifedipine 5 mg X3/d , with gradual increments to 20 mg X4/d.
Additional therapy	Oral nitrates, ß blockers, aspirin, anticoagulants, and lipid lowering drugs were permitted.

INTACT

International Nifedipine Trial on Antiatherosclerotic Therapy

(continued)

Results

There were 16 side effects in the placebo and 55 in the nifedipine group (p=0.003), and 44 vs 52 critical cardiac events (p=0.60). Cardiac mortality was 0.8% vs 2.4%, in the placebo and nifedipine groups, respectively. On the repeated angiography, ≥20% progression of stenosis in pre-existing lesions was found in 9% vs 12%, respectively, while regression of ≥20% was found in 4% and 3%, respectively. 87% vs 85% of the lesions remained unchanged (p=NS). However, new lesions in previously angiographic normal sites were found more in the placebo than nifedipine treated patients (0.82 vs 0.59 new lesions per patient, 28% reduction, p=0.034). In contrast, the mean degree of stenosis did not differ between the groups.

Conclusions

Nifedipine was associated with mild reduction of the formation of new angiographic coronary lesions. However, nifedipine was associated with more side effects and a trend towards more critical cardiac events and death.

SCRIP

The Stanford Coronary Risk Intervention Project

Title

a. Effects of intensive multiple risk factor reduction on coronary atherosclerosis and clinical cardiac events in men and women with coronary artery disease. The Stanford Coronary Risk Intervention Project (SCRIP).
b. Development of new coronary atherosclerotic lesions during a 4-year multifactor risk reduction program: the Stanford Coronary Risk Intervention Project (SCRIP).

Authors

a. Haskell WL, Alderman EL, Fair JM, et al.
b. Quinn TG, Alderman EL, McMillan A, et al.

Reference

a. Circulation 1994;89:975-990.
b. J Am Coll Cardiol 1994;24:900-908.

Disease

Coronary artery disease.

Purpose

To determine whether an intensive multifactor risk reduction program over 4 years would reduce the rate of progression of atherosclerosis.

Design

Randomized, 4 centers.

Patients

300 patients, age <75 years, with coronary artery disease (≥1 major coronary artery with 5-69% luminal stenosis that was unaffected by revascularization procedures). Patients with heart failure, pulmonary or peripheral vascular disease were excluded.

Follow-up

4 years clinical follow-up. Coronary angiography at baseline and after 4 years.

Treatment regimen	Usual care by the patients' own physician or individualized. multifactor, risk reduction program including low fat low cholesterol diet, exercise, weight loss, smoking cessation, and medications for altering lipid profile. A major goal was to decrease LDL cholesterol to <110 mg/dl and triglyceride to <100 mg/dl and to increase HDL cholesterol to >55 mg/dl.
Results	274 patients (91.3%) completed a follow-up angiogram and 246 (82%) had comparative measurements of segments with visible disease at baseline and follow-up. Intensive risk reduction resulted in highly significant improvements in various risk factors, including the lipid profile, body weight, and exercise capacity, compared with the usual care group. No change was observed in lipoprotein (a). The change in minimal luminal diameter between the 4 years and baseline angiograms was -0.024±0.066 mm/y in the risk reduction group vs -0.045±0.073 mm/y in the usual care (p<0.02). Mortality rates were similar. However, there were 25 hospitalizations in the risk reduction vs 44 in the usual care group (RR 0.61, 95% CI 0.4-0.9, p=0.05). There were 7.6% segments with new lesions in the usual care group vs 4.7% in the risk reduction group (p=0.05). New lesions were detected in 31% vs 23%, respectively (p=0.16). The mean number of new lesions/patient was 0.47 vs 0.30, respectively (p=0.06).
Conclusions	Intensive risk reduction reduced the rate of progression of luminal narrowing in coronary arteries of patients with atherosclerosis and reduced the hospitalization rate for clinical cardiac causes.

CAPRIE

Clopidogrel versus Aspirin in Patients at Risk of Ischemic Events

Title	A randomised, blinded, trial of clopidogrel versus aspirin in patients at risk of ischaemic events (CAPRIE).
Authors	CAPRIE Steering Committee.
Reference	Lancet 1996;348:1329-1339.
Disease	Atherosclerotic cardiovascular disease
Purpose	To compare the effect of clopidogrel, a new thienopyridine derivative that inhibits platelet aggregation induced by adenosine diphosphate, and aspirin in reducing the risk of ischemic stroke, myocardial infarction, or cardiovascular death in patients with atherosclerotic cardiovascular disease.
Design	Randomized, blind, multicenter.
Patients	19,185 patients with recent ischemic stroke (≤6 months), recent myocardial infarction (≤35 days), or symptomatic atherosclerotic peripheral arterial disease.
Follow-up	Average follow-up of 1.9 years (1-3 years).
Treatment regimen	Clopidogrel 75 mg X1/d or aspirin 325 mg X1/d.
Additional regimen	Use of anticoagulation or anti-platelet drugs was prohibited.

Clopidogrel versus Aspirin in Patients at Risk of Ischemic Events

(continued)

Results 21.1% vs 21.3% of the aspirin and clopidogrel-treated groups discontinued the drug early for reasons other than the occurrence of an outcome event. The rate of adverse effects was similar: rash (0.10% vs 0.26%, respectively), diarrhea (0.11% vs 0.23%), intracranial hemorrhage (0.47% vs 0.33%), and gastrointestinal hemorrhage (0.72% vs 0.52%). Neutropenia occurred in 0.10% of the clopidogrel vs 0.17% of the aspirin group, respectively. By intention to treat analysis, the clopidogrel-treated patients had an annual 5.32% risk of ischemic stroke, myocardial infarction, or vascular death compared with 5.83% among the aspirin-treated patients (relative-risk reduction of 8.7%; 95% CI 0.3-16.5; p=0.043). For patients with stroke as the inclusion criterion, the average annual event rate was 7.15% vs 7.71 with clopidegrel and aspirin, respectively (relative-risk reduction of 7.3% in favor of clopidogrel; p=0.26). For patients with myocardial infarction, annual event rates were 5.03% vs 4.84%, respectively (relative-risk increase of 3.7%; p=0.66), whereas for patients with peripheral arterial disease, the annual event rates were 3.71% vs 4.86%, respectively (a relative-risk reduction of 23.8%; 95% CI 8.9 to 36.2%; p=0.0028).

Conclusions Long-term clopidogrel therapy was more effective than aspirin in reducing the combined risk of ischemic stroke, myocardial infarction, or vascular death, especially in patients with peripheral arterial disease. Clopidogrel is as safe as medium-dose aspirin and is probably safer than ticlopidine.

The Physician's Health Study (The Beta Carotene Component)

Title	Lack of effect of long-term supplementation with beta carotene on the incidence of malignant neoplasms and cardiovascular disease.
Authors	Hennekens CH, Buring JE, Manson JE, et al.
Reference	N Engl J Med 1996;334:1145-1149.
Disease	Coronary artery disease.
Purpose	To evaluate the long term effect of beta carotene supplementation on mortality and morbidity.
Design	Randomized, double-blind, placebo-controlled, multicenter
Patients	22,071 U.S. male physicians, 40 to 84 years old at entry, with no history of cancer, myocardial infarction, stroke, or transient cerebral ischemia.
Follow-up	An average of 12 years (11.6 to 14.2 years).
Treatment regimen	Randomization to one of 4 groups: 1. Aspirin 325 mg on alternate days + ß carotene 50 mg on alternate days; 2. Aspirin + ß carotene placebo; 3. Aspirin placebo + ß carotene; 4. Both placebo.

The Physician's Health Study (The Beta Carotene Component)

(continued)

Results

The randomized aspirin component of the study was terminated early in 1988 because there was a statistically significant 44% reduction in the risk of first myocardial infarction with aspirin ($p<0.001$). The ß carotene component continued as planned. By the end of 11 years of follow-up, 80% of the participants were still taking the drug medication, 78% of the study drugs were still being taken by the ß carotene patients, whereas 6% of the placebo group were taking supplemental ß carotene. There were no early or late differences in overall mortality, the incidence of malignancy or cardiovascular disease between the groups. Myocardial infarction occurred in 468 vs 489 patients in the ß carotene and placebo groups, respectively ($p=0.50$), stroke in 367 vs 382 patients ($p=0.60$), death from cardiovascular disease in 338 vs 313 patients ($p=0.28$), and the number of any of the major cardiovascular endpoints 967 vs 972 patients ($p=0.90$). There were no major side effects associated with ß carotene supplementation.

Conclusions

Supplementation with ß carotene for 12 years was not associated with either benefit or harm concerning mortality, incidence of malignancy, or cardiovascular morbidity.

CARET

The Beta-Carotene and Retinol Efficacy Trial

Title	Effects of a combination of beta carotene and vitamin A on lung cancer and cardiovascular disease.
Authors	Omenn GS, Goodman GE, Thornquist MD, et al.
Reference	N Engl J Med 1996;334:1150-1155.
Disease	Cardiovascular disease.
Purpose	To assess the efficacy of beta-carotene and retinol (Vitamin A) supplementation to reduce incidence of cancer and mortality rate from cancer and cardiovascular disease.
Design	Randomized, double-blind, placebo-controlled, multicenter.
Patients	18,314 men and women, 45 to 74 years of age, who were smokers, former smokers, or workers exposed to asbestos.
Follow-up	mean length of follow-up, 4.0 years.
Treatment regimen	Patients were randomized to a combination of 30 mg/d ß carotene and retinyl palmitate 25,000 IU/d, or placebo.
Additional therapy	Supplemental intake of vitamin A was restricted to <5500 IU/d. Beta carotene supplementation was prohibited.

CARET

The Beta-Carotene and Retinol Efficacy Trial

(continued)

Results

The ß carotene-retinol treated patients had higher incidence of lung cancer than the placebo group (5.92 vs 4.62 cases/1000 person-year; a relative risk 1.28; 95% CI 1.04 to 1.57; p=0.02). Total mortality was 14.45 vs 11.91 deaths per 1000 person-year, respectively; relative risk 1.17; 95% CI 1.03 to 1.33; p=0.02). The ß carotene-retinol group had a relative risk of cardiovascular mortality of 1.26 (95% CI 0.99 to 1.61). On the basis of these findings, the randomized trial was terminated prematurely.

Conclusions

Supplementation of ß carotene and retinol for an average of 4 years in high risk patients (smokers, and workers exposed to asbestos) had no benefit on the incidence of cancer and on mortality from cardiovascular causes and cancer. Supplementation of ß carotene and retinol may have had an adverse effect on the incidence of lung cancer and mortality.

The Iowa Women's Health Study

Title	Dietary antioxidant vitamins and death from coronary heart disease in postmenopausal women.
Authors	Kushi LH, Folsom AR, Prineas RJ, et al.
Reference	N Engl J Med 1996;334:1156-1162.
Disease	Coronary artery disease.
Purpose	To asses whether dietary intake of antioxidants is related to mortality from coronary artery disease.
Design	Prospective cohort study.
Patients	34,386 postmenopausal women, 55-69 years of age.
Follow-up	7 years.
Treatment regimen	The study evaluated the intake of vitamins A, E, and C from diet and supplements.
Results	In analyses adjusted for age and dietary calorie intake, an inverse correlation was found between vitamin E consumption and cardiovascular mortality. This association was especially significant in the subgroup of women who did not consume vitamin supplements (n=21,809; relative risks from lowest to highest quintile of vitamin E intake, 1.0, 0.68, 0.71, 0.42, and 0.42; p for trend=0.008). After adjustment for confounding variables, this association remained significant (relative risks 1.0, 0.70, 0.76, 0.32, and 0.38; p for trend=0.004). Multivariate analysis suggested no association between supplemental vitamin E intake and risk of death from coronary artery disease. Intake of vitamins A and C was not associated with the risk of mortality from coronary heart disease.

Conclusions In postmenopausal women the intake of vitamin E from food, but not from supplements, is inversely associated with mortality rate from coronary heart disease. This may suggest that vitamin E consumed in food is a marker for other dietary factors associated with the risk of coronary heart disease. By contrast, intake of vitamins A and C, either from diet or from supplements, was not associated with lower mortality from coronary disease.

CHAOS

Cambridge Heart Antioxidant Study

Title	Randomised controlled trial of vitamin E in patients with coronary disease: Cambridge heart antioxidant study (CHAOS).
Authors	Stephens NG, Parsons A, Schofield PM, et al.
Reference	Lancet 1996;347:781-786.
Disease	Coronary artery disease.
Purpose	To determine whether treatment with high dose α-tocopherol (Vitamin E) would reduce the incidence of myocardial infarction and cardiovascular death in patients with ischemic heart disease.
Design	Randomized, double blind, placebo-controlled, single-center.
Patients	2002 patients with angiographically proven coronary artery disease. Patients with prior use of vitamin supplements containing vitamin E were excluded.
Follow-up	Median follow-up 510 days (range 3 to 981 days).
Treatment regimen	α-tocopherol (Vitamin E) 400 or 800 IU/d or placebo.

CHAOS

Cambridge Heart Antioxidant Study

(continued)

Results

Plasma α-tocopherol levels were increased in the actively treated group (from baseline mean 34.2 μmol/L to 51.1 μmol/L with 400 IU/d and to 64.5 μmol/L in the 800 IU/d), but remained the same in the placebo group (32.4 μmol/L). Treatment with α-tocopherol did not affect serum cholesterol. α-tocopherol therapy significantly reduced the risk of cardiovascular death and myocardial infarction. Non-fatal myocardial infarction occurred in 1.4% vs 4.2% of the α-tocopherol and placebo group, respectively (relative risk (RR) 0.23; 95% CI 0.11 to 0.47; $p<0.001$). However, cardiovascular mortality was similar (2.6% vs 2.4%, respectively; RR 1.18; 95% CI 0.62 to 2.27; $p=0.61$). Treatment was well tolerated. All cause mortality was 3.5% vs 2.7% ($p=0.31$). Only 0.55% of the patients discontinued therapy because of side effects. There was no significant difference between the placebo and α-tocopherol groups in occurrence of side effects.

Conclusions

α-tocopherol therapy in patients with coronary artery disease reduced the rate of non-fatal myocardial infarction. However, there was no effect on total or cardiovascular mortality.

11. Ongoing Clinical Trials

During the last years numerous studies have been conducted on various cardiovascular subjects. In the previous chapters we described some of the major studies that have already been completed and published in the medical literature. Nevertheless, several other important studies are still ongoing, or their preliminary results have been published as abstracts.

In this chapter we shall review some of these ongoing studies:

1. Acute Myocardial Infarction

GUSTO II

Intravenous Heparin Versus Recombinant Hirudin for Acute Coronary Syndromes

Reference	Circulation 1994;90:1631-1637.
Disease	Acute myocardial infarction, unstable angina pectoris.
Purpose	To compare the efficacy and safety of recombinant hirudin with heparin in acute coronary syndromes.
Design	Randomized, double blind, multicenter.
Patients	Adult patients, with chest discomfort and ECG changes, within 12 h of onset of symptoms, and no contraindications to thrombolytic therapy or heparin.
Follow-up	30 day clinical follow-up.
Treatment regimen	Thrombolytic therapy with either tissue plasminogen activator or streptokinase for patients with ST segment elevation. Patients were randomized to heparin or hirudin infusion for 72-120 h.
Remarks	GUSTO-2A was terminated prematurely after 2564 patients were enrolled due to higher rates of hemorrhagic stroke in the hirudin treated patients. GUSTO 2B was continued with lower doses of hirudin. Preliminary data presented at the American College of Cardiology meeting 1996 suggested that hirudin had no major treatment benefit over heparin on 30 day mortality but a small reduction in recurrent myocardial infarction rate.

PARAGON

Delaying and preventing ischemic events in patients with acute coronary syndromes using the platelet glycoprotein IIb/IIIa inhibitor lamifiban

Reference	J. Am. Coll. Cardio. 1997; 29 (Suppl A); 409A
Disease	Unstable angina, non Q-wave myocardial infarction
Purpose	To determine the incidence and timing of 30 day reinfarction or infarction and in-hospital refractory ischemia in patients receiving low or high dose lamifiban with or without heparin versus standard therapy
Design	Randomized, multicenter
Patients	2282 patients with unstable angina or non Q wave myocardial infarction
Follow-up	30 days
Treatment regimen	Low dose lamifiban vs. high dose lamifiban, with or without heparin, versus standard therapy - heparin alone
Remarks	Low dose lamifiban with and without heparin delayed and prevented infarction/reinfarction and ischemic events compared to other groups.

CAPTURE

Reduction of recurrent ischemia with abciximab during continuous ECG-ischemia monitoring in patients with unstable angina refractory to standard treatment (CAPTURE)

Reference	J. Am. Coll. Cardiol. 1997; 29 (Suppl A); 367A.
Disease	Unstable angina
Purpose	To determine the incidence of recurrent ischemia in patients receiving abciximab or placebo in addition to standard therapy for unstable angina.
Design	Randomized
Patients	Patients with unstable angina (332 in this subset)
Follow-up	6 hours of 12 lead ECG ischemia monitoring after start of treatment
Treatment regimen	Abciximab vs. placebo regimen
Remarks	5 abciximab patients (3%) compared to 15 placebo patients (9%) had ≥ 3 ST episodes. Abciximab reduced total duration and degree of ST segment abnormality (p<.01 - .02). Authors concluded that abciximab reduced total ischemic burden in patients with unstable angina.

PAMI-2

Primary Angioplasty in Myocardial Infarction-2

Reference	Circulation 1995;92:693-694.
Disease	Acute myocardial infarction.
Purpose	To evaluate the effectiveness of both early discharge (third day) in low-risk patients and intra-aortic balloon pumping in high-risk patients with acute myocardial infarction undergoing primary angioplasty.
Design	Randomized.
Patients	471 low-risk and 437 high-risk patients with acute myocardial infarction undergoing primary angioplasty.
Follow-up	In-hospital events.
Treatment regimen	Early discharge (third day) vs 5-7 days in low-risk patients. Intra-aortic balloon pumping in high-risk patients.

PAMI STENT PILOT STUDY

Safety and feasibility of primary stenting in acute myocardial infarction - In-hospital and 30 day results of the PAMI Stent Pilot Trial

Reference	J. Am Coll Cardiol 1997;29 (Suppl A); 389A.
Disease	Acute Myocardial Infarction
Purpose	To determine safety and feasibility of primary stenting in acute myocardial infarction
Design	nonrandomized, multicenter
Patients	300 acute myocardial infarction patients. Average age 61; 27% female.
Follow-up	1 month
Treatment	PTCA followed by stents. ReoPro in 5%; IC urokinase in 1%. Most pts. discharged on aspirin and/or ticlopidine.
Remarks	97% stented patients achieved TIMI 3. In hospital death 0.4%; recurrent MI 1.3%. At 1 month 207 pts eligible for follow up had 0 death, 0 reinfarction rates. Authors commented that these short-term results appeared better than their previous experience with primary PTCA for acute myocardial infarction.

GRAMI TRIAL

Coronary stents improved hospital results during coronary angioplasty in acute myocardial infarction: Preliminary results of a randomized controlled study (GRAMI Trial)

Reference	J. Am. Coll. Card. 1997; 29 (Suppl A); 221A
Disease	Acute Myocardial Infarction
Purpose	To determine if GRII (Cook Inc) stents can improve outcome in patients undergoing angioplasty during acute myocardial infarction.
Design	Randomized
Patients	Preliminary report of 65 patients randomized to primary PTCA (n=25) versus stent (n=40) for acute myocardial infarction. Patients underwent angiography predischarge. No difference in age, sex, previous MI, Killip class.
Follow-up	In hospital, ongoing.
Treatment	Primary PTCA vs stent. Stent patients received IV heparin for 48 hours, aspirin, ticlopidine.
Remarks	Technical failure or death occurred in 24% of PTCA patients and 0% of stent patients. Authors conclude that stents as a primary therapy of myocardial infarction improved this composite endpoint.

GUSTO III

Global Use of Strategies to Open Occluded Arteries III

Reference	Presentations at the 1997 American College of Cardiology Meetings (Topol E. et al.)
Disease	Acute Myocardial Infarction
Purpose	To compare the outcomes of treating patients with acute myocardial infarction with tissue plasminogen activator, alteplase (t-PA) versus recombinant plasminogen activator, reteplase (r-PA)
Design	Randomized, multicenter
Patients	15,000 acute myocardial infarciton patients
Preliminary Results	The risk of death at 30 days was 7.22% in patients given t-PA and 7.43% in those given r-PA. The incidence of hemorrhagic strokes was 0.88% for t-PA and 0.91% for r-PA. r-PA did not appear better than t-PA for these endpoints.

2. Unstable Angina

IMPACT-II

Integrelin to Manage Platelet Aggregation to Combat Thrombosis

Reference	Circulation 1995;91:2151-2157. Circulation 1995;92:697.
Disease	Unstable angina.
Purpose	To evaluate the efficacy of integrelin, a platelet glycoprotein IIb/IIIa receptor blocker, as an adjunct to coronary intervention.
Design	Randomized, double blind, placebo-controlled, multicenter.
Patients	4010 patients who underwent coronary angioplasty or atherectomy.
Follow-up	30 days.
Treatment regimen	Patients were randomized to either integrelin 135 μg/kg bolus + 0.5 μg/kg/min infusion for 24 h; integrelin 135 μg/kg bolus + 0.75 μg/kg/min infusion, or placebo. All patients received aspirin and procedural heparin.
Remarks	Preliminary data were presented at the 1995 European Society of Cardiology meeting. At 24 hours, both Integrelin groups had fewer outcome events (high-dose 7.0%, low dose 6.8%) than placebo (9.3%, $p<0.01$). 30-day event rate was 9.5% in the Integrelin treated groups vs 11.4% in the placebo (p=NS). There was no difference in the complication rates.

PRISM

Platelet Receptor Inhibitor for Ischemic Syndrome Management

Reference	Presentation at the 1997 American College of Cardiology Meetings (White H. et al).
Disease	Coronary artery disease. Chest pain due to unstable angina, non-Q wave myocardial infarction.
Purpose	To determine outcomes of a 48 hour infusion of the platelet glycoprotein (GP) IIb/IIa receptor blocker tirofiban, versus heparin.
Design	Randomized, double blind
Patients	Patients with chest pain due to unstable angina, non Q wave myocardial infarction. 1,616 patients received heparin, 1,615 received tirofiban.
Follow-up	30 days.
Treatment regimen	48 hour infusion of tirofiban compared to heparin.
Preliminary Results	At 48 hours, the composite endpoint (death, new myocardial infarction, refractory ischemia) was 3.8% in tirofiban group, 5.9% in heparin group (p=0.007). At 30 days death was 2.3% in tirofiban group versus 3.6% in heparin group (p=0.02).

PRISM-PLUS

Platelet Receptor Inhibittion for Ischemic Syndrome Management in Patients Limited by Unstable Signs and Symptoms (PRISM-PLUS)

Reference	Presentation at the 1997 American College of Cardiology Meetings (Theroux P. et al).
Disease	Coronary Artery Disease. Unstable angina, non-Q wave myocardial infarction.
Purpose	To determine effectiveness of tirofiban in high risk patients with unstable angina or non Q wave myocardial infarction in context of use of aspirin, heparin, and interventional cardiology.
Patients	High risk patients with unstable angina, non Q wave myocardial infarction. 773 patients received heparin plus tirofiban; 797 received heparin alone.
Follow-up	30 days.
Treatment regimen	48 hour infusion of tirofiban plus heparin versus heparin alone.
Preliminary Results	At 7 days the composite endpoint (death, myocardial infarction, refractory ischemia) was 12.9% in tirofiban plus heparin versus 17.9% with heparin alone (p=0.004). At 30 days the composite endpoint was 18.5% with tirofiban and 22.3% with heparin. There was a trend toward more bleeding with tirofiban plus heparin than heparin alone.

VANQWISH

Veterans Affairs Non-Q Wave Infarction Strategies In-Hospital

Reference	Presentation at the 1997 American College of Cardiology Meetings (Boden W. et al).
Disease	Non-Q wave myocardial infarction.
Purpose	To compare outcomes in patients with non Q wave myocardial infarctions rendomized to early invasive strategy versus conservative management.
Design	Randomized.
Patients	920 patients.
Follow-up	At least 12 months.
Treatment regimen	Early invasive strategy: Coronary angiography and revascularization. Early conservative strategy: Radionuclide ventriculogram, thallium stress test.
Preliminary Results	At time of hospital discharge there were 6 deaths with early conservative therapy versus 21 in invasive group. After hospital discharge there were 53 deaths in the conservative group versus 59 in invasive group. Invasive group had all cause mortality that was 30% greater long term compared to conservative group. Average length of hospital stay was 8.2 in conservative group versus 9.5 in invasive group. Authors suggest that initial conservative management strategy be used in patients with non-Q wave myocardial infarction.

FLARE

The Fluvastation Angioplasty Restenosis Trial

Reference	Presentation at the 1997 American College of Cardiology Meetings (Serruys PW et al).
Disease	Coronary artery disease.
Purpose	To determine effect of treatment with the cholesterol-lowering agent fluvastatin on outcome after percutaneous transluminal coronary angioplasty.
Design	Randomized.
Patients	1054 patients.
Follow-up	9 months.
Treatment regimen	Fluvastatin 2 weeks before and for 26 weeks after angioplasty.
Preliminary Results	No difference in the primary endpoint of angiographically-determined change in minimal lumen diameter. Incidence of death and myocardial infarction was reduced in the fluvastatin group versus placebo group (1.5% versus 4%). Fluvastatin reduced low density lipoprotein cholesterol by 33-37%. Although lipid lowering did not affect restenosis rates it did reduce death plus myocardial infarction rate.

3. Hypertension

ALLHAT

Antihypertensive and Lipid Lowering Treatment to Prevent Heart Attack Trial

---

Reference	J National Med Assoc 1995;87:627-629.
Disease	Hypertension.
Purpose	1. To assess whether antihypertensive therapy with amlodipine, lisinopril, doxazosin or chlorthalidone is associated with reduced incidence of fatal coronary heart disease or non-fatal myocardial infarction. 2. To determine whether pravastatin therapy for moderately hypercholesterolemic patients ≥60 years old will reduce mortality.
Design	Randomized, open label, multicenter.
Patients	40000 patients, ≥60 years old, with hypertension are expected to be recruited. Patients with fasting LDL cholesterol 120-189 mg/dl and triglyceride <350 mg/dl will be eligible for the cholesterol lowering substudy.
Follow-up	7 years.

LIFE STUDY

Losartan Intervention for Endpoint Reduction in Hypertension

Disease	Hypertension
Purpose	To compare the effects of losartan and atenolol on cardiovascular mortality and morbidity in patients with hypertension.
Design	Randomized, triple-blind, controlled.
Patients	8300 patients, aged 55-88 years, with hypertension and ECG documented LVH. Patients with prior myocardial infarction, heart failure or stroke will be excluded.
Follow-up	4 years or more.
Treatment regimen	2 week placebo initiation period. Active therapy for 4 years. Randomization to losartan + placebo or placebo + atenolol in daily 50 mg doses. Hydrochlorothiazide and additional agents may be added to provide blood pressure control.

HOT

The Hypertension Optimal Treatment

Reference	1. Blood Pressure 1993;2:62-68. 2. Blood Pressure 1994;3:322-327. 3. Blood pressure 1995;4:313-319.
Disease	Hypertension.
Purpose	1. To determine what is the optimal therapeutic goal for diastolic blood pressure (≤90, ≤85 or ≤80 mmHg) for patients with hypertension in order to prevent cardiovascular morbidity and mortality. 2. To assess the efficacy of low dose aspirin in reduction of cardiovascular mortality and morbidity in hypertensive patients.
Design	Randomized, open label, multicenter.
Patients	19,196 patients, 50-80 years old, with diastolic blood pressure 101-115 mmHg.
Follow-up	>2 years.
Treatment regimen	1. Felodipine 5 mg/d. If blood pressure is not controlled, additional therapy according to 4 more steps is given: low dose ACE inhibitor or ß blocker; the felodipine dose is increased to 10 mg; the dose of the additional drug is increased; an alternative drug or hydrochlorothiazide is added. 2. Aspirin 75 mg/d or placebo.

CAPPP

The Captopril Prevention Project

Reference	1. J Hypertens 1990;8:985-990. 2. Am J Hypertens 1994;7:82S-83S.
Disease	Hypertension.
Purpose	To compare the effectiveness of conventional therapy with diuretics and or ß blockers vs captopril in patients with hypertension regarding cardiovascular mortality.
Design	Randomized, open label, placebo-controlled, multicenter.
Patients	10800 patients, 25-66 years old, with diastolic blood pressure >100 mmHg.
Follow-up	5 years.
Treatment regimen	Captopril 50 mg/d or conventional therapy (ß blockers or diuretics).

Syst-Eur

Systolic Hypertension-Europe

Reference	1. Aging 1991;3:287-302. 2. Clin Exper Hypertens 1993;15:953-966. 3. J Human Hypertension 1993;7:265-271. 4. J Human Hypertension 1993;7:411-412. 5. J Hypertens 1994;12:1035-1039.
Disease	Hypertension.
Purpose	To evaluate the effectiveness of antihypertensive therapy in prevention of cardiovascular complications in patients >60 years old with isolated systolic hypertension.
Design	Randomized, double blind, placebo-controlled, multicenter.
Patients	Aim 3000 patients, >60 years old, with sitting systolic blood pressure 160-219 mmHg, and diastolic blood pressure <95 mmHg.
Follow-up	6 years.
Treatment regimen	Nitrendipine 10-40 mg/d (if necessary combined with enalapril 5-20 mg/d, and hydrochlorothiazide 12.5-25 mg/d) or matching placebo. Goal of systolic blood pressure: <150 mmHg, with a reduction of at least 20 mmHg.
Remarks	Initial reports on the first 941 patients suggested that in the placebo group the average fall in sitting systolic blood pressure over the first six months was 5±18 mmHg, and in the diastolic blood pressure 0±9 mmHg. In patients receiving active therapy the decrease in blood pressure was 19±18 and 5±9 mmHg, respectively. From 9 months onwards, 15% of the placebo vs 40% of the active treatment group had attained goal blood pressure (p=0.001). Fewer patients remained on monotherapy in the placebo than in the active treatment group (p<0.001), and in the placebo group the second and third line medications were started earlier (p<0.001). Study medication was discontinued in 9 of the placebo-treated patients and in 29 patients assigned to active therapy (p<0.001).

PRESERVE

Prospective Randomized Enalapril Study Evaluating Regression of Ventricular Enlargement

Reference	Am J Cardiol 1996;78:61-65.
Disease	Hypertension.
Purpose	To compare the efficacy of enalapril and nifedipine GITs to reduce left ventricular mass and to normalize the Doppler echocardiographic ratio of early to late mitral inflow flow velocities in hypertensive patients.
Design	Randomized, double blind, parallel-group, multicenter.
Patients	480 patients, ≥50 years old, with ≥140 mmHg systolic blood pressure if on anti-hypertensive therapy, or ≥150 systolic blood pressure if unmedicated, and/or ≥90 mmHg diastolic blood pressure, and echocardiographic LV mass >116 g/m^2 in men and >104 g/m^2 in women. Patients with left ventricular ejection fraction <0.40 or evidence of severe valvular heart disease or coexisting cardiomyopathy will be excluded.
Follow-up	1 year with clinical follow-up and repeated echocardiogram at baseline, 6 and 12 months.
Treatment regimen	Enalapril 10-20 mg/d or nifedipine GITs 30-60 mg/d. In cases where maximum dose is reached and further blood pressure control is needed, hydrochlorothiazide 25 mg, and then atenolol 25 mg will be added.

STONE

Shanghai Trial of Hypertension in the Elderly

Reference	Cardiovasc Drugs Ther 1996;10:467-468.
Disease	Hypertension.
Purpose	To compare the efficacy of nifedipine with placebo in patients with hypertension.
Design	Single-blind.
Patients	1632 patients, 60-79 years old, with blood pressure ≥160/90 mmHg.
Follow-up	32 months.
Treatment regimen	Randomization to placebo or nifedipine slow-release retard 10 mgX2/d. If the blood pressure remained above 159/90, captopril and/or thiazide was added.
Remarks	Initial report suggested that systolic blood pressure was reduced by nifedipine, but diastolic blood pressure was only slightly changed. The relative risk of stroke was reduced to 0.43. The relative risk of malignant tumors was 0.24. Mortality tended to fall in the nifedipine group in those who did not receive combination therapy (p=0.06). However, mortality was not changed in those who received combination therapy (p=0.2). Final results have not been published yet.

STOP Hypertension 2

Swedish Trial in Old Patients with Hypertension 2

Reference	Blood Pressure 1993;2:136-141
Disease	Hypertension
Purpose	A prospective interventional trial of "newer" versus "older" treatment alternatives in old patients with hypertension. STOP Hypertension 1 showed that among elderly men and women (aged 70-84) treated for hypertension (with a beta blocker - atenolol, metroprolol or pindolol - and diuretic hydrochlorothlazide plus amiloride) comapred to placebo, that there was a 47% reduction in stroke morbidity and mortality, 40% reduction in all cardiovascular endpoints and 43% reduction in total mortality with therapy (Lancet 1991;338:1281-1285). STOP Hypertension 2 will compare the effect of older drugs (beta blockers and diuretics) to the newer alternative (calcium channel blockers-isradipine and felodipine) and ACE-inhibitors (enalapril and lisinopril) on cardiovascular mortality.
Design	Prospective, randomized, open, blinded endpoint evaluation.
Patients	Over 6600 hypertensive patients ages 70-84 years with supine BP> or = 180/105 mmHg.
Follow-up	4 years.
Treatment regimen	Diuretic - beta blocker regimen against either ACE-inhibitor (enalapril. lisinopril) or calcium blockers (isradipine, felodipine).

4. Congestive Heart Failure

MACH -1

Mortality Assessment in Congestive Heart Failure

Reference	Clin Cardiol 1997;20:320-326
Disease	Congestive heart failure
Purpose	To assess whether addition of mibefradil, a non-voltage-regulated T-channel calcium blocker, to standard therapy for heart failure will reduce mortality in patients with heart failure
Design	Randomized, placebo controlled, double-blind, parallel-group, multicenter
Patients	2,400 patients, ≥20 years old, with left ventricular ejection fraction <35% and left ventricular end diastolic diameter >60 mm, and symptomatic heart failure (NYHA class II-IV), who are stabe on therapy comprising of loop diuretics and angiotensin converting enzyme inhibitors. Digoxin and other vasodilators are permitted.
Follow-up	2-3 years.
Treatment regimen	Mibefradil 50 or 100 mg/d or matching placebo

5. Prevention of Progression of Coronary Artery Disease

QUIET

The Quinapril Ischemic Event Trial

Reference Blood Pressure 1992;1(Suppl 4):11-12.

Disease Coronary artery disease.

Purpose To evaluate the role of quinapril, an ACE inhibitor, on the development of ischemic events and progression of atherosclerosis in patients with coronary artery disease.

Design Randomized, placebo controlled, multicenter.

Patients 1900 patients with coronary artery disease, <75 years old, with left ventricular ejection fraction ≥40%, a serum LDL cholesterol ≤165 mg/dl, a blood pressure <160/95 mmHg

---

Follow-up 3 year clinical follow-up. In 500 patients- repeated coronary angiography.

Treatment regimen Quinapril 20 mg/d or placebo.

INDEX

INDEX

(continued)

INDEX

(continued)

INDEX

(continued)

INDEX

(continued)

NOTES

NOTES

NOTES

NOTES

NOTES

NOTES

NOTES

NOTES

NOTES

NOTES

NOTES

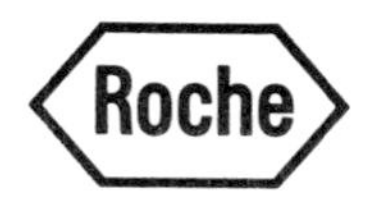

POSICOR®

(mibefradil dihydrochloride)

TABLETS

DESCRIPTION: POSICOR® (mibefradil dihydrochloride) is a selective T-type calcium channel ion influx inhibitor.

Mibefradil dihydrochloride is a pure enantiomer and belongs to the class of tetralol calcium antagonists. Its chemical name is (1S, 2S)-2-[2[[3-2-benzimidazoyl) propyl] methylamino] ethyl]-6-fluoro-1,2,3,4-tetrahydro-1-isopropyl-2-naphthylmethoxyacetate dihydrochloride, its empirical formula is $C_{29}H_{38}FN_3O_3 \cdot 2HCl$, its molecular weight is 568.56, and its structural formula is:

·2HCl

Mibefradil dihydrochloride is a white to off-white crystalline powder. It is readily soluble in water.

In addition to the active ingredient mibefradil dihydrochloride, each tablet contains the following inactive ingredients: lactose anhydrous, corn starch, polyvinylpyrrolidone, talc, sodium stearyl fumarate, hydroxypropyl methylcellulose, ethyl cellulose, triacetin and titanium dioxide, with synthetic yellow iron oxide (50 mg tablet) and synthetic red iron oxides (100 mg tablet).

CLINICAL PHARMACOLOGY: ***Mechanism of Action:*** At therapeutic concentrations, mibefradil blocks both the T-type (low-voltage) and L-type (high-voltage) calcium channels, with greater selectivity for T-type channels, in contrast to benzothiazepine, dihydropyridine, and phenylalkylamine calcium antagonists, which at therapeutic concentrations block only the L-type channels. The binding site of mibefradil is different from that of the dihydropyridines.

The contractile processes of cardiac muscle and vascular smooth muscle are dependent upon the movement of extracellular calcium ions into these cells through specific ion channels. In vitro, mibefradil selectively inhibits calcium ion influx across cell membranes of cardiac and vascular smooth muscle with a pronounced dependence on membrane potential. The dose and concentration ranges for vasodilation were lower than, and clearly distinct from, the ranges where a decrease in cardiac contractility was observed. This was observed both in vivo and in vitro and in both normal animals and in animal models of heart failure. Although in in vitro tissue preparations mibefradil was negatively inotropic at high concentrations, negative inotropic effects could be demonstrated in intact animals only at very high doses, well outside the therapeutic range.

Mibefradil does not induce reflex tachycardia, but rather causes a slight reduction in heart rate.

Serum calcium concentration was not affected by mibefradil.

Hypertension: Mibefradil is a peripheral arterial vasodilator that acts directly on vascular smooth muscle to cause a reduction in peripheral vascular resistance, and thereby a reduction in blood pressure.

Chronic Stable Angina Pectoris: The precise mechanism by which mibefradil reduces angina has not been fully elucidated but is thought to involve reduction in heart rate, total peripheral resistance (afterload), and double product (heart rate x systolic blood pressure) at any given level of exercise, resulting in a decrease in cardiac workload and myocardial oxygen demand.

Pharmacokinetics and Metabolism: After oral administration of POSICOR, peak plasma levels of mibefradil are reached within 1 to 2 hours after administration. Bioavailability of a single oral dose of mibefradil within the therapeutic range was 70%. The proportion of mibefradil metabolized before reaching the systemic circulation (first-pass metabolism) is reduced after chronic dosing and bioavailability is about 90% at steady-state. The presence of food has no effect on rate and extent of absorption of mibefradil. Mean elimination half-life following chronic dosing is 17 to 25 hours. During once-daily dosing, steady-state conditions are reached within 3 to 4 days. Plasma AUCs are proportional to dose in the therapeutic range.

DISTRIBUTION: Volume of distribution at steady-state (V_{ss}) ranges from 130 to 190 L. Mibefradil is highly bound to plasma proteins (≥99% at therapeutic concentrations), principally to alpha$_1$-acid glycoprotein.

METABOLISM: Metabolism of mibefradil is mediated by two pathways: esterase catalyzed hydrolysis of the ester side chain to yield an alcohol metabolite and cytochrome P450 (3A4) catalyzed oxidation. After chronic dosing, the oxidative pathway becomes less important and the plasma level of the alcohol metabolite of mibefradil increases. In animal models the pharmacological effect of this alcohol metabolite was about 10% of the parent compound. At steady-state, plasma concentrations of the metabolite exceed those of parent mibefradil after 100 mg doses.

EXCRETION: After metabolic inactivation, mibefradil is excreted into the bile (75%) and urine (25%). Less than 3% of mibefradil is excreted unchanged into the urine. No clinically relevant influence of demographic factors (age, race, gender, body weight) on clearance has been found.

SPECIAL POPULATIONS: Congestive Heart Failure: There is no evidence for a change in the pharmacokinetics of mibefradil in patients with congestive heart failure.

Hepatic Insufficiency: No clinically relevant change in the pharmacokinetics of mibefradil in patients with impaired liver function was observed after single doses of 100 mg POSICOR. As mibefradil is completely metabolized and eliminated mainly via the biliary route, however, monitoring of blood pressure and heart rate is advised when administering POSICOR to patients with severe hepatic impairment.

Chronic Renal Failure: Pharmacokinetics of mibefradil are unchanged in patients with chronic renal failure. Mibefradil is not removed by dialysis.

Gender/Race: No clinically relevant difference in the pharmacokinetics of mibefradil was observed between either men and women or between blacks and non-blacks.

Pediatrics: No studies have been conducted in pediatric patients.

Geriatrics: Population kinetics in 315 patients (151 ≥ 65 years) indicated that there was no change in the pharmacokinetics of mibefradil with age.

DRUG INTERACTIONS: See PRECAUTIONS.

Pharmacodynamics: The plasma concentrations of mibefradil are predictive of its pharmacological effects.

Hemodynamics: Following administration of mibefradil to patients with hypertension, POSICOR produces a dose-related and plasma concentration-related reduction of supine, sitting and standing blood pressure, without postural dysregulation. These decreases in blood pressure following multiple dosing are accompanied by a slight increase in cardiac output with a small, dose-dependent decrease in heart rate. The magnitude of the blood pressure reduction depends on initial blood pressure; the higher the initial blood pressure, the greater the effect.

Blood pressure lowering effect is maintained for 24 hours following chronic oral administration of POSICOR. Normotensive subjects experienced no clinically relevant change in blood pressure after chronic dosing with 50 mg to 100 mg mibefradil. The reduction in heart rate seen with mibefradil depends on the initial heart rate; the lower the initial heart rate, the smaller the effect. The concentration effect relationship was not influenced by demographic factors (age, race, gender).

Electrophysiology: Mibefradil affects the sinus and atrioventricular nodes, resulting in a slight dose-dependent slowing of heart rate and a small increase in PR interval. In placebo-controlled clinical trials in patients with hypertension or chronic stable angina pectoris, the mean decreases in heart rate were about 5 and 9 beats per minute (bpm) with 50 mg (N=279) and 100 mg (N=285) of POSICOR, respectively. In these patients, the mean increase in PR interval was 3.3 msec (50 mg) and 9.7 msec (100 mg). The increases, compared to placebo, of the rate of first-degree AV block (PR interval > 200 msec) were 1.1% at 50 mg, 7.4% at 100 mg and 9.1% at 150/200 mg. The rates of sinus bradycardia (heart rate < 45 bpm) were 0.7% at 50 mg, 1.4% at 100 mg and 3.8% at 150/200 mg. In 2636 patients with hypertension or chronic stable angina pectoris, treatment with POSICOR 50 mg or 100 mg was rarely associated with second-degree AV block (6 patients, 0.2%) and there were no reports of third-degree AV block.

The effects of mibefradil on the conduction system were evaluated in 71 patients in a placebo-controlled trial. Mibefradil was administered IV at doses that produced plasma concentrations seen following oral administration of mibefradil at 50 mg and 100 mg. In this study, mibefradil slightly lengthened the corrected sinus node recovery time and AH interval and raised the Wenckebach point. Atrial effective and functional refractory periods, AV node functional and effective refractory periods and the conduction time in the His-Purkinje system and ventricular tissue were not affected.

Mibefradil causes dose-related flattening of the T wave and an increase in the voltage of the U wave. The U wave can sometimes become so large that it merges with the flattened T wave, and the resulting pattern has sometimes been misread (by both automated electrocardiographic interpreters and clinicians) as QTc prolongation.

The exact definition of this phenomenon is arbitrary. Changes sufficient to be misread as QTc prolongation in clinical trials did not occur at the therapeutic doses of 50 mg or 100 mg of mibefradil but were observed in 1% of patients who received 150 mg and 5.4% of patients who received 200 mg, both of which are above the recommended doses. Similar patterns have been seen in subjects treated with high and supratherapeutic doses of diltiazem and verapamil.

The addition of POSICOR to chronic beta-blocker treatment was evaluated in both hypertensive and chronic stable angina pectoris patients (195 patients) and was associated with changes in heart rate and PR interval similar to those seen in patients treated with mibefradil alone. There were no cases of second- or third-degree AV block in these patients. In 44 angina patients treated with POSICOR and beta-blockers, no acute withdrawal effects, such as worsening of angina or palpitations, were seen upon beta-blocker discontinuation. However, care should be taken when combining POSICOR with beta-blockers (see WARNINGS), particularly when the heart rate is already slow.

The combination of POSICOR and digoxin was not associated with an additional prolongation of PR time beyond the effect of POSICOR alone.

Effects in Hypertension: The antihypertensive effects of POSICOR were demonstrated in four placebo-controlled, double-blind, randomized trials conducted for 4 to 14 weeks, three in patients receiving no other treatment and one in patients still hypertensive while receiving 25 mg of hydrochlorothiazide. These involved 1123 patients with hypertension (933 on POSICOR and 190 on placebo). Once-daily administration of 50 mg and 100 mg was consistently associated with clinically and statistically significant reductions in both systolic and diastolic blood pressure. The mean differences from placebo in systolic/diastolic blood pressure at trough (24-hours postdose), for the 50 mg and 100 mg doses were about 7-11/5-7 and 7-10/9-11 mmHg, respectively. The antihypertensive effect of POSICOR was present in the sitting, standing and supine positions. The antihypertensive effect was not associated with reflex tachycardia, but rather a slight decrease in heart rate. The blood pressure was controlled over the 24-hour dosing interval, with little difference between trough and peak effect (trough to peak ratio >75%). A modest effect was seen on Day 1, and the full antihypertensive effect was reached within 1 to 2 weeks.

Long-term antihypertensive effects were demonstrated in two 4-month, randomized, placebo-controlled withdrawal studies involving 221 patients on mibefradil. Blood pressure returned to approximately pretreatment levels in 4 weeks. Thus, there was no tolerance (loss of efficacy) observed on long-term administration. Additionally, no rebound increase in blood pressure was seen on discontinuation of POSICOR.

The antihypertensive effects of POSICOR were similar regardless of race, gender, body weight, history of diabetes mellitus or history of coronary artery disease. POSICOR was effective in lowering high blood pressure in patients with chronic renal failure complicated by systemic hypertension. Additive antihypertensive effects have been observed in clinical trials where POSICOR was combined with diuretics, ACE inhibitors and beta-blockers.

Effects in Chronic Stable Angina Pectoris: The antianginal and antiischemic efficacy of POSICOR was demonstrated in five placebo-controlled, double-blind, randomized trials, involving 870 patients with chronic stable angina pectoris, 564 on POSICOR and 306 on placebo. Once-daily administration of 100 mg was associated with statistically significant increases in all exercise test parameters, in all studies, but the effect of 50 mg was smaller and less consistent. The increases in symptom-limited exercise duration at trough (24-hours postdose) for POSICOR 50 mg and 100 mg were about 20 seconds (seen in two of three studies) and about 50 seconds (in all three studies), respectively. In these studies, POSICOR also significantly delayed the time to onset of angina during exercise and, in a pooled analysis, decreased the rate of anginal attacks and nitroglycerin consumption reported by the patients. Additionally, POSICOR significantly delayed the onset of ischemia (persistent 1mm ST segment depression) during exercise in all placebo-controlled studies. These antianginal and antiischemic effects were associated with a dose-dependent mean decrease in double product for any given level of exercise (heart rate x systolic blood pressure), mainly due to a decrease in heart rate.

Long-term improvements in exercise test parameters were demonstrated in a 4-month, randomized, placebo-controlled withdrawal study involving 102 patients on mibefradil. Thus, there was no tolerance (loss of efficacy) observed on long-term administration. Additionally, no rebound increase in anginal symptomatology was seen on discontinuation of POSICOR.

POSICOR® (mibefradil dihydrochloride)

The antianginal effects of POSICOR were similar regardless of gender, race, body weight or history of hypertension, diabetes mellitus, myocardial infarction, PTCA or CABG. Improvements in all exercise test parameters and anginal symptomatology were observed in three placebo-controlled, double-blind, randomized clinical trials in which POSICOR was added to therapy with beta-blockers or long-acting nitrates.

INDICATIONS AND USAGE: *Hypertension:* POSICOR is indicated for the treatment of hyper tension. POSICOR can be used alone or in combination with other antihypertensive agents.

Chronic Stable Angina Pectoris: POSICOR is indicated for the treatment of chronic stable angina pectoris. POSICOR can be used alone or in combination with other antianginal drugs.

CONTRAINDICATIONS: POSICOR is contraindicated in patients who:

1. Have sick sinus syndrome or second- or third-degree AV block, without a pacemaker;
2. Have a known sensitivity to mibefradil;
3. Are concurrently receiving terfenadine, astemizole, cisapride, lovastatin or simvastatin (see WARNINGS and PRECAUTIONS).

WARNINGS: ***Suppression of Sinoatrial Node Activity:*** **Use of mibefradil has been associated with slowing or complete suppression of sinoatrial node activity. The supervening junctional rhythms have often been slow (as slow as 30 to 40 bpm). Many of the reports have incorrectly identified the adverse event as complete AV block. The reports have been most common in the elderly, mainly in association with the concomitant use of beta-blockers. Care should be taken when combining POSICOR with beta-blockers, particularly when pretreatment sinus rate is below 55 bpm, and this combination should be avoided in the elderly when pretreatment sinus rate is below 55 bpm (see PRECAUTIONS). In patients with low heart rates, use of any combination of agents that can slow the sinus node or affect the AV node (eg, beta-blockers, digitalis, and the calcium-channel blockers mibefradil, diltiazem, and verapamil) should in general be undertaken only after careful consideration, as such combinations can unmask underlying sick sinus syndrome. Use of POSICOR in patients with sick sinus syndrome without a pacemaker is contraindicated (see CONTRAINDICATIONS).**

Electrocardiographic Changes: As described in the CLINICAL PHARMACOLOGY section, mibefradil may cause dose-related changes in the appearance of the electrocardiographic T and U waves. These changes may interfere with measurement of the QTc interval. Some drugs (eg, quinidine, sotalol) are sometimes monitored by following the QTc interval on serial electrocardiograms, in order to reduce the risk of torsades de pointes and other malignant arrhythmias. When mibefradil is coadministered with these drugs, it may be difficult to utilize serial electrocardiograms for this purpose.

Interaction Resulting in HMG-CoA Reductase Inhibitor-Induced Rhabdomyolysis: **Mibefradil inhibits the action of CYP 450 3A4. When this enzyme is inhibited, plasma concentrations of those drugs that are metabolized by CYP 450 3A4 may become elevated, sometimes by more than an order of magnitude (see PRECAUTIONS).**

Rhabdomyolysis is a known rare adverse effect of all of the HMG-CoA reductase inhibitors (the "statin" cholesterol-lowering agents).

The statins are not identically metabolized:

- **Lovastatin and simvastatin are dependent on CYP 450 3A4 for their metabolic clearance. Among patients receiving simvastatin and mibefradil there have been reported cases of rhabdomyolysis. These events appear to reflect an incidence of rhabdomyolysis higher than that seen during treatment with simvastatin alone. Because of the metabolic similarities of lovastatin and simvastatin, coadministration of POSICOR with either of these two drugs is contraindicated.**
- **Atorvastatin** and **cerivastatin** are biotransformed by CYP 450 3A4 to active and inactiv metabolites. Also, only small changes in HMG-CoA reductase inhibitor activity have bee seen in studies where atorvastatin and cerivastatin were combined with erythromycin (less potent CYP 450 3A4 inhibitor than mibefradil). Nevertheless, until there is more infor mation on the coadministration of CYP 450 3A4 inhibitors (including mibefradil) with ato vastatin and cerivastatin, **coadministration of either of these two drugs with POSICO should generally be avoided.**
- Fluvastatin and pravastatin are not significantly metabolized by CYP 450 3A4; no clinicall important interaction with mibefradil is anticipated. Therefore, no specific dose adjustme of fluvastatin or pravastatin is recommended with coadministration of POSICOR.

Drug Interactions — Cyclosporine/Tacrolimus and HMG-CoA Reductase Inhibitors: Th calcineurin immunosuppressants tacrolimus (FK-506) and cyclosporine are metabolized b CYP 450 3A4, so their blood levels rise (in the case of cyclosporine, about twofold) whe POSICOR is coadministered; dose adjustment may be necessary. Because the immunosuppressants themselves inhibit a drug-transport system that participates in the excretion o HMG-CoA reductase inhibitors, elevated levels of the immunosuppressants can cause additional elevations in the blood levels of any of the HMG-CoA reductase inhibitors. **Use of POSICOR should be avoided in patients also receiving both a calcineurin immunosuppressant and an HMG-CoA reductase inhibitor.**

PRECAUTIONS: ***General:*** POSICOR inhibits cytochrome P450 2D6 and 3A4 and can interact with many concomitant drugs, increasing their plasma concentrations (see *Drug Interactions* and WARNINGS).

Hypotension: Although hypotension, postural hypotension and syncope have been only rarely associated with POSICOR, and are not clearly more common than with placebo, caution should be exercised when administering POSICOR, particularly to patients with severe aortic stenosis.

Use in Patients With Congestive Heart Failure: Acute hemodynamic studies in a small number of patients with ischemic heart disease with or without impaired cardiac function treated with POSICOR have not demonstrated negative inotropic effects, nor was POSICOR associated with reflex tachycardia or an increase in neurohormones. Long-term studies in patients with moderate to severe (NYHA III, IV) heart failure have not been carried out. As with all calcium antagonists, caution should be exercised when treating patients with heart failure or compromised ventricular function.

Patients With Hepatic Failure: Since mibefradil is extensively metabolized by the liver, caution should be exercised when administering POSICOR to patients with severe hepatic impairment.

Cardiac Conduction: As described under CLINICAL PHARMACOLOGY, POSICOR slows sinus and AV node conduction, sometimes resulting in abnormally low heart rates; 0.7% and 1.4% of patients had heart rates below 45 bpm on 50 mg and 100 mg, respectively. Therefore, patients with a pretreatment heart rate below 55 bpm should be followed closely. Treatment with POSICOR has rarely been associated with second-degree AV block, 0.2% of patients on doses of 50 mg to 100 mg. One case of third-degree AV block occurred in clinical trials at a 150 mg dose of POSICOR. Care should be taken when combining POSICOR with beta-blockers, particularly when pretreatment sinus rate is below 55 bpm, and this combination should be avoided in the elderly when pretreatment sinus rate is below 55 bpm (see WARNINGS).

Drug Interactions: *EFFECTS OF OTHER DRUGS ON MIBEFRADIL PHARMACOKINETICS:* No clinically relevant changes in pharmacokinetics of mibefradil have been seen in specific studies when mibefradil was coadministered with enalapril, atenolol, metoprolol, theophylline and cimetidine.

EFFECTS OF MIBEFRADIL ON THE PHARMACOKINETICS OF OTHER DRUGS: INTERACTIONS WITH DRUGS METABOLIZED BY CYTOCHROME P450 ENZYMES: In vitro results indicate that some isozymes of the cytochrome P450 enzyme system, including 2D6, 1A2, and 3A4, are inhibited in the presence of mibefradil or its metabolites. Coadministration of POSICOR with drugs metabolized by these isozymes may result in increased plasma concentrations of these drugs.

DRUGS METABOLIZED BY CYTOCHROME P450 2D6: A subset (about 7%) of the white population and 1% and 2% of Orientals and blacks, respectively, have reduced activity of the drug-metabolizing isozyme cytochrome P450 2D6 (debrisoquine hydroxylase). Such individuals are referred to as "poor metabolizers" of such drugs as dextromethorphan, the type 1C antiarrhythmics propafenone, flecainamide and mexiletine, some beta-blockers and tricyclic antidepressants (particularly those with high first-pass effect, ie, desipramine and imipramine). Poor metabolizers have higher than expected plasma concentrations of such drugs when given in usual doses. Depending on the fraction of the drug metabolized by cytochrome P450 2D6, the increase in plasma concentration may be small or quite large. POSICOR, like several other drugs, inhibits the activity of this isozyme and can make previously normal metabolizers resemble poor metabolizers. Concomitant use of POSICOR with drugs metabolized by cytochrome P450 2D6 may require dose adjustment of the other drugs.

Tricyclic Antidepressants: Imipramine and desipramine have been shown to have substantial (seven- to eightfold) increases in AUC when CYP 450 2D6 metabolism is inhibited; concomitant use of tricyclic antidepressants with POSICOR would require substantial dose adjustment of the tricyclic antidepressant.

Drugs Metabolized by Cytochrome P450 3A4: POSICOR and/or its metabolites also inhibit the activity of cytochrome P450 3A4, an enzyme responsible for the metabolism of many drugs, including quinidine, short-acting benzodiazepines, most calcium-channel blockers, terfenadine, astemizole and cisapride. POSICOR may increase plasma concentrations of coadministered drugs that are primarily metabolized by the cytochrome P450 3A4 enzyme system and may consequently increase or prolong their therapeutic and adverse effects. Therefore, unless otherwise specified, dosage adjustment of these drugs may be necessary. For drugs that can cause serious adverse effects if concentration is increased, concomitant use with POSICOR should be avoided (see CONTRAINDICATIONS).

The following drug interactions have been identified involving mibefradil and other drugs metabolized by the cytochrome P450 system:

HMG-CoA Reductase Inhibitors: See CONTRAINDICATIONS and WARNINGS.

Cyclosporine and Tacrolimus: See WARNINGS.

Terfenadine: Coadministration of terfenadine (metabolized by CYP 450 3A4) with POSICOR in healthy subjects led to elevated plasma concentrations of terfenadine up to 40 ng/mL with twice-daily dosing of 60 mg terfenadine, resulting in a 12% increase in mean QTc interval. Since QTc prolongation due to elevated plasma concentrations of terfenadine can be associated with life-threatening cardiac dysrhythmias and death, coadministration of POSICOR with terfenadine is contraindicated (see CONTRAINDICATIONS).

Astemizole and Cisapride: Although there are no specific studies of interaction of mibefradil with these drugs, substantial inhibition of their metabolism would be expected. Since elevated plasma concentrations of astemizole and cisapride can be associated with life-threatening cardiac dysrhythmias, their use with mibefradil is contraindicated. One such case has been observed in a patient receiving cisapride and concomitant mibefradil.

Quinidine: In healthy volunteers, elevations in peak quinidine plasma concentrations (15% to 19%) and AUC (50%) were found during coadministration of single doses of quinidine with POSICOR 50 mg and 100 mg, but the active metabolite of quinidine was markedly reduced. No clinically relevant pharmacodynamic interactions were observed.

Metoprolol: Coadministration of POSICOR with metoprolol (metabolized by CYP 450 2D6) in healthy subjects resulted in a twofold increase in peak plasma concentrations of total (R- and S-enantiomeric) metoprolol and about four- to fivefold increase in AUC. Elimination half-life increased from 3 hours to 7 to 8 hours. The increase in the pharmacologically more active S-isomer, however, is only about 30%, so that little pharmacologic effect or effect on cardioselectivity would be expected with concomitant POSICOR.

OTHER INFORMATION: In clinical studies, POSICOR has been administered without apparent harm with commonly used drugs including diuretics, ACE inhibitors, nonsteroidal anti-inflammatory drugs, long-acting nitrates, sublingual nitroglycerin, oral hypoglycemics, fibrate lipid-lowering agents, conjugated estrogens, antibiotics and antithrombotics.

SPECIFIC INTERACTION STUDIES: In specific studies, no clinically relevant interactions have been observed between the recommended doses of POSICOR and enalapril, atenolol or cimetidine. Despite in vitro evidence of inhibition of CYP 450 1A2, no pharmacokinetic interaction was observed with theophylline, a CYP 450 1A2 substrate. In healthy volunteers, small elevations in digoxin peak plasma levels (20% to 30%) were found during coadministration with POSICOR 50 mg and 100 mg, but trough plasma levels were unchanged in these volunteers and in patients with congestive heart failure.

PROTEIN BINDING: Mibefradil is highly protein bound (99.5%), mainly to alpha$_1$-acid glycoprotein (95%). Therefore, it will not displace drugs which bind to serum albumin, such as warfarin, phenytoin and digoxin.

Information for Patients: Patients should be instructed to take POSICOR whole and not to crush or chew the tablet. Patients should inform their physicians if they are pregnant or plan to become pregnant or are breastfeeding. Patients should be informed that light-headedness or fatigue can occur and that these symptoms should be reported to a physician.

Carcinogenesis, Mutagenesis and Impairment of Fertility: Mibefradil was not mutagenic in the Ames microbial mutagenicity test with or without metabolic activation, in the microbial test with *E. coli* or in Chinese hamster V79 cells. No genotoxicity was observed in a test of unscheduled DNA synthesis in rat primary hepatocytes, and no chromosomal damage was observed in a test of human peripheral blood lymphocytes treated in vitro or in an in vivo micronucleus test.

A decrease in mating incidence and a prolongation of time to mating was observed when male and female rats were treated with mibefradil dihydrochloride at a daily dose of 39 mg mibefradil/kg (approximately three times the maximum recommended human dose [MRHD] on a mg/m^2 basis) prior to and during the mating period. For those females successfully mated at this dose, there was a decrease in fetuses/dam observed at caesarean section or pups/dam at natural delivery, findings associated with both a decrease in number of corpora lutea per dam (evidence of a decrease in ovulation) and an increase in preimplantation loss (ovulations not resulting in implants).

Oral gavage administration of mibefradil dihydrochloride to male mice for up to 95 weeks and to female mice for up to 104 weeks at doses up to 65 mg mibefradil/kg/day (about three times the MRHD of 100 mg mibefradil/day on a mg/m^2 basis) revealed no evidence of a carcinogenic effect of mibefradil. When administered in the feed of rats at doses of 35 mg mibefradil/kg/day (about three times the MRHD on a mg/m^2 basis) for up to 104 weeks, an increased incidence of squamous cell carcinoma of the oral cavity was observed. A similar association was observed when another rat study was conducted with similar doses of mibefradil administered by gavage. The latter study, which evaluated diet as a risk factor for the oral cavity tumors, demonstrated that the carcinogenic effect of mibefradil was dependent on the aggressiveness (in terms of producing severe periodontitis) of the diet employed combined with class-related gingival overgrowth. No tumors were observed when mibefradil was administered to rats fed a less aggressive diet associated with much lower levels of periodontitis.

Pregnancy: Pregnancy Category C. Developmental toxicity studies have been conducted in rats and rabbits. In rabbits, no adverse effects on development were seen with doses up to 35 mg mibefradil/kg/day (approximately seven times the MRHD on a mg/m^2 basis). In rats there was an increased incidence of fetuses with cardiovascular abnormalities at 39 mg/kg/day (approximately three times the MRHD). Skeletal and visceral defects have been observed following the administration of other calcium antagonists to pregnant rodents or rabbits. There are no adequate and well-controlled studies in pregnant women. POSICOR should be used during pregnancy only if the potential benefit justifies the potential risk to the fetus.

Labor and Delivery: Dystocia and/or prolongation of pregnancy, which was associated with uterine prolapse, stillbirths and neonatal mortality, was observed to occur when mibefradil dihydrochloride was administered to pregnant rats, during the expected time of parturition, at 13 or more mg mibefradil/kg/day (13 mg/kg/day is approximately equal to the MRHD on a mg/m^2 basis). Calcium-channel blocking agents have been shown to inhibit uterine contraction in rats, rabbits and humans, presumably by inhibition of Ca^{++} influx in the myometrium.

POSICOR should be avoided during the time of expected labor and during parturition.

Nursing Mothers: When mibefradil was administered to lactating rats, their milk attained mibefradil concentrations two to five times greater than those in their serum. If mibefradil enters human milk in similar quantities, then a human infant ingesting such milk would (scaling directly by weight) be expected to develop serum mibefradil levels somewhat less than those of the mother. On the other hand, mibefradil levels have not been measured in human milk. The pharmacokinetics and pharmacodynamics of mibefradil in human infants have not been studied, and neonates have been reported to be disproportionately sensitive to some other calcium-channel blockers. Administration of mibefradil should therefore be avoided, if possible, in lactating women who continue to nurse.

Pediatric Use: Safety and effectiveness of POSICOR in pediatric patients have not been established.

Geriatric Use: In clinical studies, POSICOR was shown to be effective and well-tolerated in elderly patients with hypertension or chronic stable angina pectoris. However, concomitant use of POSICOR and beta-blockers should be avoided in the elderly when pretreatment sinus rate is below 55 bpm (see WARNINGS).

ADVERSE REACTIONS: POSICOR has been evaluated for safety in 3430 patients (2194 with hypertension, 1236 with chronic stable angina pectoris). In general, treatment with POSICOR was well tolerated at doses up to 100 mg daily. Most adverse reactions associated with POSICOR were transient and of mild or moderate intensity. In placebo-controlled clinical trials, the rate of discontinuation of POSICOR (50 mg and 100 mg) due to adverse reactions was similar to that of placebo. Discontinuation due to dizziness was the only reason for premature withdrawal that was more common on mibefradil than on placebo. In the pooled placebo-controlled hypertension and chronic stable angina pectoris trials that studied doses of 50 mg/day and 100 mg/day, the incidence of adverse experiences present in at least 1% of patients treated with the 100 mg dose and more common on that dose than on placebo were:

	Placebo	**POSICOR**	
	(N=283)	**50 mg (N=279)**	**100 mg (N=285)**
Headache	6%	3%	8%
Leg Edema	3%	1%	4%
Rhinitis	0%	3%	3%
Abdominal Pain	1%	1%	2%
Light-headed Feeling	0%	1%	3%
Dyspepsia	1%	1%	2%

The following adverse experiences were also present in >1% of patients treated with the 100 mg dose but occurred at a frequency equal to or less than placebo: allergic reaction, angina pectoris, dizziness, fatigue, flushing, influenza, palpitations, upper respiratory tract infection and vomiting/nausea.

The following adverse experiences occurred in a dose-related manner in placebo-controlled trials over a dose range of 50 mg to 150 mg: dizziness, dyspepsia, flushing, leg edema, rhinitis and vomiting/nausea.

There were no clinically important differences in the effect of POSICOR on adverse experience rates based on age, gender or race.

In the 2636 patients treated with POSICOR (50 mg or 100 mg) in controlled or uncontrolled trials, the following adverse experiences, whether drug related or not, occurred at a frequency greater than 0.5% or occurred at a lower rate but were potentially important:

Autonomic Nervous System: increased sweating, orthostatic complaints, postural hypotension, syncope

POSICOR® (mibefradil dihydrochloride)

Body as a Whole: generalized weakness, trauma

Cardiovascular: bradycardia, cardiac failure, chest pain nonspecific, hypotension

Central and Peripheral Nervous System: paresthesia

Gastrointestinal: constipation, diarrhea, flatulence, gastroenteritis, rectal hemorrhage

Hearing and Vestibular: ear buzzing, otitis

Immunologic: angioedema

Musculoskeletal: arthritis, back pain, chest pain, muscle cramps, pain of extremities, sprains and strains

Psychiatric: anxiety, depression, insomnia

Reproductive, Male: impotence

Respiratory: bronchitis, coughing, dyspnea, nasal congestion, pharyngitis, sinusitis

Skin and Appendages: exfoliative dermatitis, rash

Urinary System: urinary tract infection

Vision: conjunctivitis

Electrocardiographic Changes: Treatment-emergent ECG changes that clearly occurred in a dose-related manner in the placebo-controlled trials were bradycardia (heart rate < 45 bpm): 0.7% (50 mg) and 1.4% (100 mg) and first-degree AV block: 3.6% (50 mg) and 8.4% (100 mg). In the 2636 patients treated with POSICOR (50 mg or 100 mg) in controlled or uncontrolled trials, second-degree AV block was recorded in 0.2% of the patients. Junctional rhythm has been reported in association with sinus node dysfunction and/or sinus arrest and third-degree AV block has been reported (see WARNINGS).

POSICOR therapy has not been associated with clinically significant changes in routine laboratory tests. No clinically relevant changes were noted in hematology parameters, serum potassium, sodium, calcium, glucose, plasma lipids, uric acid, urea nitrogen, creatinine or liver function tests.

OVERDOSAGE: At present there has been no experience with single doses >350 mg or multiple doses >250 mg. Doses higher than these might cause excessive peripheral vasodilation with marked hypotension, bradycardia and/or high-degree AV block. If a patient is suspected of having taken an overdose, continuous ECG monitoring and repeated blood pressure measurements should be instituted. Should hypotension occur, cardiovascular support including elevation of the extremities and the judicious administration of fluids should be initiated. If hypotension remains unresponsive to these measures, administration of vasopressors (such as phenylephrine) should be considered with attention to circulating volume and urine output. Intravenous calcium gluconate may help to reverse the effects of calcium antagonists. As mibefradil is highly bound to plasma proteins, it cannot be removed by dialysis.

Bradycardia and high-degree AV block may be treated with atropine, isoproterenol and cardiac pacing.

DOSAGE AND ADMINISTRATION: The recommended doses of POSICOR are 50 mg and 100 mg once daily. The larger dose is, on average, more effective. Doses above 100 mg offer little or no additional benefit and induce a greater rate of adverse reactions. POSICOR can be taken with or without food. Tablets should be swallowed and not chewed or crushed.

Hypertension: The recommended initial dose of POSICOR is 50 mg once daily. Titration to 100 mg once daily should be based on blood pressure response; the full effect of a given dose level is generally seen after 1 to 2 weeks. The same dosage recommendations apply for all populations, including elderly patients and patients with chronic renal failure. However, caution should be exercised in patients with severe hepatic impairment.

Chronic Stable Angina Pectoris: The recommended initial dose of POSICOR is 50 mg once daily. Titration to 100 mg once daily should be based on therapeutic response. The same dosage recommendations apply for all populations, including elderly patients and patients with chronic renal failure. However, caution should be exercised in patients with severe hepatic impairment.

Coadministration With Other Antihypertensive and/or Antianginal Drugs: POSICOR has been safely administered with diuretics, ACE inhibitors, long-acting nitrates and sublingual nitroglycerin.

Administration in Subpopulations: POSICOR has been used safely in patients regardless of demographic factors (age, race, gender, body weight) and common concomitant diseases, such as chronic renal failure, chronic obstructive pulmonary disease and diabetes mellitus.

HOW SUPPLIED: POSICOR is supplied as biconvex, hexagonal tablets, available in bottles and Tel-E-Dose® packages as follows:

	50 mg	100 mg
color	pale yellow	light orange
engraving	ROCHE POSICOR 50	ROCHE POSICOR 100
bottle of 100	NDC 0004-0080-01	NDC 0004-0081-01
bottle of 300	NDC 0004-0080-27	---
Tel-E-Dose® of 100	NDC 0004-0080-49	NDC 0004-0081-49

Storage Conditions: Store at 15° to 30°C (59° to 86°F) in tight containers as defined in USP/NF.

Roche Pharmaceuticals

Roche Laboratories Inc.
340 Kingsland Street
Nutley, New Jersey 07110-1199

25993568-1297
25829852-1297

Revised: December 1997
Printed in USA